MANAGING YOUR DOCTOR

MANAGING YOUR DOCTOR

THE SMART PATIENT'S GUIDE TO GETTING EFFECTIVE AFFORDABLE HEALTHCARE

———

Patrick Neustatter MD

Edited by Eric Mohrman

ISBN: 1508802580
ISBN 13: 9781508802587
Library of Congress Control Number: 2015903906
CreateSpace Independent Publishing Platform
North Charleston, South Carolina

ACKNOWLEDGMENTS

PARTICULAR THANKS TO ERIC MOHRMAN, who acted as editor, mentor, and guide to help keep me on track and from getting too weird/esoteric/medical.

Particular thanks also to Dr. Steve Mussey, M.D. for allowing me to use his wacky but poignant cartoons he's drawn over the years for the local Free Lance-Star newspaper.

Thanks and apologies to wife Paula for putting up with me spending years sitting at my computer, beating my brains out, wanting absolute quiet in the household.

And thanks to many others who encouraged me and gave sage advice on writing and process and were willing to read through different parts of the draft to give direction--particularly Anita Bihovsky and my sister, Angela Neustatter.

TABLE OF CONTENTS

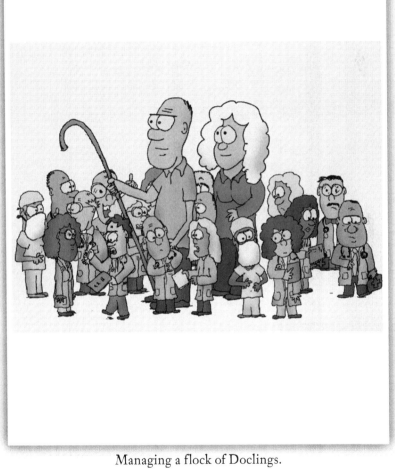

Managing a flock of Doclings.

INTRODUCTION

———

"Doctors are men who prescribe medicines
of which they know little,
To cure diseases of which they know less,
In human beings of whom they know nothing."

- Voltaire

WITH HIS SCATHING CRITICISM AND wicked humor, Voltaire long ago perfectly expressed why you need this healthcare guide.

Your doctor isn't necessarily the entirely competent, omnipotent god he (and maybe you) believes he is. And you—the sort of human being about which your doctor knows nothing—need to embrace the role of empowered, assertive, involved patient to help fill the gaps in what your doctor knows and oversee your care.

Maybe this strikes a chord. Maybe you were treated like some unknown species, misdiagnosed, or left anguishing for years with a constellation of symptoms no one could figure out. Maybe you received treatments not because they were best for you, but because they were the most advertised, convenient, or profitable. Maybe you haven't found a doctor who is the perfect match for you and your illness. Maybe you're tired of waiting so long to get appointments only to be hurried out the door by a doctor who doesn't even seem to listen to a word you say. Maybe your healthcare has left you with insurmountable medical bills...

The antidote is information. That's where I come in.

This book advises you on getting the right doctor, diagnosis, information, treatment, price, and even—strange as it may sound—the right death. It concludes with a look at where healthcare is headed and how we can get the future right, too.

It's about becoming an emancipated, proactive patient, no longer content to sit, cap in hand, submissively leaving every decision to paternalistic doctors who believe management of your health isn't your business.

Before I lose you (if you're like me, you're glibly sampling a few paragraphs to decide if this book's for you), I assure you this isn't another whimsical compilations of heartwarming stories interspersed with eye-roll humor compiled by some science writer, medical correspondent, or ghostwriter.

This guide provides solidly useful information. It's based on the condensed wisdom of a zigzag forty-year career path ending with twenty-four years as a no-frills, down-to-earth family physician (one of the "grunts" of the medical world) in the U.S.

Though trained at one of the most prestigious medical schools in England (Guy's Hospital), I am not some ivory tower academic incapable of expressing things in an understandable way. I've given this guide a light touch, with some editorializing (I call it "a guide book with an attitude") and anecdotes, partly to appeal to that voyeuristic tendency referred to as "peeking around the curtain" by Jim Hall, the recently retired medical correspondent for my local newspaper.

As an Englishman, I'm expected to hide my light under a bushel and not make audacious claims. Still, I like to think I'm the right person to navigate you through the dangers, discomforts, and expenses of the tortuous road to good healthcare.

FROM ROOTS TO RETIREMENT

Some kind of engagement with medicine seemed inevitable for me. Born in England to an eccentric psychiatrist father and a committed philanthropist mother, I became the fifth generation of doctors.

The conviction that you should be liberated and have charge of your healthcare probably comes from my schooling at a wacky, self-governing "progressive," do-as-you-like institution. Dartington Hall School in Devon was modeled after the archetype, Summerhill, started by my step-grandfather, A.S. Neill, and my paternal grandmother, his first wife.

I learned self sufficiency, fair play, contentment, curiosity, and how to be a happy, healthy child, though probably more from extracurricular activities like working on the school farm, forestry, and arts and crafts more than schooling. My not-so-polished academic skills made for a stressful transition to the Dickensian wards of the venerable Guy's Hospital at London Bridge, founded in the 1700s by Sir Thomas Guy with a fortune made from importing bibles. The establishment's culture appeared frozen in the era of the great names of medicine, after whom the dingy wards were named: Astley Cooper, Richard Bright, Thomas Addison, etc.

I passed six years as a dweeby, anxious medical student in a confrontational atmosphere of derisive, condescending consultants/attendings who delighted in belittling and ridiculing (shades of the teacher in Pink Floyd's *The Wall*). My academic inferiority gave me a lifelong resentment of "knowledgism," a term I coined for regurgitating factoids. It's good for passing exams, but takes no account of important but unquantifiable, more nebulous doctoring characteristics, like common sense, problem-solving skills, listening skills, and compassion.

After graduation, I went through the zigzag phase, including jobs in orthopedics, the ER, anesthetics, general practice, and medical editing. I also traveled a lot, sometimes working (in mission hospitals in Zimbabwe, Haiti, Ecuador, and a brief stint as a flying doctor in Broken Hill, Australia), sometimes not, as when traveling "the Hippy Trail" to India in the mid-70s with a fellow doctor and old school chum. We took a VW minibus through places like Iran, Afghanistan, and the Khyber Pass, where I guess even a bunch of naive, drug-crazed travelers wouldn't go these days.

Feeling the need to settle, I was persuaded to come to the U.S. by my first-wife-to-be. I moved to her stomping grounds in New York, where I experienced another shock: immersion in that in-your-face New York culture. It met me up front and personal in a Family Medicine residency program at the University Hospital of SUNY at Stony Brook on Long Island.

Finally a full-fledged family physician, I joined a multispecialty practice just north of Fredericksburg, Virginia and experienced the satisfaction of getting to know my patients more intimately than ever before. I considered myself more a friend of the family with medical knowledge than their doctor.

As part of this practice, I was a preceptor for University of Virginia students, entitling me to the grandiose attribution of "Visiting assistant professor of family medicine," and perhaps serving as a small nod to my competence. I delighted in showing them "the real world" of high-productivity primary care medicine (which one student described as "drinking from a fire hose").

Family life took a back seat and I finished up with an unhappy taste of the American domestic legal system and divorce. It made for scheduling nightmares when I lived alone, trying never be on call on kids' nights or working kids' weekends. It was well worth it, though, bringing me much closer to daughters Tegan and Alexis.

The 30 acres of rural splendor/jungle we lived on suffered the neglect of my "survivalist gardening" until I remarried, to Paula, with her green thumb and enthusiasm for making the place look its best.

Besides medicine, a second familial proclivity that afflicts me is a compulsion to write. It puts me in mind of Anton Chekhov, a physician by trade, who said, "Literature is my mistress, medicine my lawful wedded wife."

I think there's a genetic component here as well. The most famous writer in the family is my father's maternal aunt, Ethel Florence Lindsay Richardson (pen name Henry Handle Richardson). Her trilogy, *The Fortunes of Richard Mahoney*, is a vivid picture of my great grandfather's life as an Irish doctor who emigrated to Australia during the gold rush, traveling into the bush on horseback or buggy for days at a time for house calls (and his distress at patients' reluctance to pay combined with his being too proper to ask). The work is a sort of synthesis of the writing and medical facets of the family.

Writing was more than just my mistress for two years, when I worked as medical editor of the now-defunct *Medical News* in London. I've continued as a blowhard with a monthly column in the Healthy Life section of my local newspaper, *The Free Lance-Star*, and blogging as a politically incorrect, outspoken curmudgeon in Dr. Gagg's Diary (my alter ego).

The final chapter of my career path—the one that allowed me to indulge the insane amount of time it's taken to put this guide together—was stepping off the treadmill. With some remorse, I abandoned my suffering patients and tried to retire in 2010. "Tried" because of a slight compromise in becoming part-time volunteer medical director for the local Lloyd Moss Free Clinic for the medically indigent (of whom I find there are many in this rich and prosperous country).

A VENDOR-ORIENTATED CHALLENGE TO THE CONSUMER

After twenty-four years in the trenches, beating my head against the wall as a primary care doctor in the U.S. with something of an outsider perspective, I'm well aware of many challenges American healthcare consumers—and their doctors—face.

I see the differences between the privately run, free-enterprise, entrepreneurial U.S. system and the single-payer, government-run British National Health Service. Incidentally, I am not a refugee from the NHS, as everyone assumes of any British doctor in the U.S. On the contrary, at the risk of being seen as a pinko wingnut, I think nationalized healthcare would be a good thing for America.

The fee-for-service payment system ("medicine by the yard," as the wags call it) provides an incentive to "do everything" and over-treat, in contrast to the NHS, where payment is capitated, incentivizing the opposite. Yes, people often wait a long time for nonessential treatments like getting varicose veins stripped or a hip replaced, but medical bills aren't bankrupting people. Under the current U.S. system, the country spends twice as much or more per head on healthcare than other industrialized nations ($8,233 in the U.S., as opposed to $3,433 in the U.K. in 2010, for example).

In contrast to the U.K., I see a fairly prevalent attitude in America that healthcare isn't something that should be a government-sponsored entitlement. For some reason, though, education, defense, roads, law enforcement, parks, and a whole lot of other things are.

Healthcare consumers in the U.S. are subject to the caprices of for-profit corporations, which have tilted the playing field to their advantage. For example, they've persuaded Congress to ban international import of cheap drugs (medicines cost Americans about twice as much as people in other industrialized countries; in some, like Canada, there are government checks on drug prices); Medicare has been refused the ability to negotiate "economy of scale" drug discounts like the VA does; and direct-to-consumer advertising for drugs is permitted (New Zealand being the only other country in the world where this is the case). The corporations have also managed to prevent tort reform on malpractice to reduce expensive defensive medicine and to deal a deathblow to the Patient-Centered Outcomes Research Institute's Comparative Effectiveness ranking of "best practices" that was meant to be part of the Affordable Care Act.

"The reality [is] that our largest consumer product by far—one-fifth of our economy—does not operate in a free market", and sellers have "overwhelming leverage," notes Steven Brill in his great article, "Bitter Pill: Why Medical Bills Are Killing Us," in *TIME* of March 2013.

The for-profit industry in the U.S. protects its market, keeping costs and charges a closely guarded secret, likened to trying to buy a car when no one will tell you the price. Hospitals use a completely capricious and incomprehensible "chargemaster" billing schedule with no basis in what things cost, as discussed in more detail in the chapter *Getting the Right Price*. Usually, those who feel the brunt of this insane pricing are those who can least afford it: the uninsured and underinsured.

This entrepreneurial system has also led to problems with a mandated innovation, electronic health records. Multiple vendors jealously guard and promote their own systems rather than sharing, which would greatly benefit patient care. And the innumerable insurance companies with their different policies, regulations, and billing systems make for a wildly inefficient system.

Further consumer discombobulation comes from insane charge discrepancies between hospitals, even closely neighboring ones. For example, in figures recently released for the first time by the Centers for Medicare and Medicaid Services, admission for chronic obstructive pulmonary disease (COPD) costs $7,044 in one hospital and a cool $99,690 at another less than 30 miles away.

Hospitals and medical practices are increasingly being bought up by corporations and turned into widget factories where the bottom line is the primary concern, and overall, healthcare generates huge profits. Hospitals do business worth $2.5 trillion annually.

Forbes reports four of the country's ten most profitable industries are healthcare related. Financial information company Sageworks reports an industry-wide profitability of 14.1 percent. The international research company McKinsey & Co. reports outpatient emergency room care averages an operating profit margin of 15 percent and non-emergency outpatient care averages 35 percent. These are some of the highest industry profit margins in the country.

Doctors, unless they're also investors (a lot are), do not share in this bounty. Their annual incomes have dropped in recent periods, with primary care doctors like pediatricians and family physicians earning an average of about $150,000.

Those profitable industries include things like medical device manufacturing and pathology labs. But, although a bit past its zenith, the pharmaceutical industry takes the cake with profits at 16.3 percent, according to *Kaiser Health News*, about double that of the average American corporation.

This all adds to the skyrocketing cost of healthcare that currently consumes 17.6 percent of the U.S. GDP, with the prediction to rise to 25 percent by 2025 (as compared to the average for OECD countries of 9.5 percent), driving up health insurance premiums. Many people are oblivious to the costs, though, thanks to the attitude of "price doesn't matter, the insurance company's paying."

Currently, movements toward different ways of paying—by capitation or results rather than per service, for example—are catching on, but they have a long way to go.

The ability of this prosperous industry to arrange things to their advantage comes from access to large quantities of that highly influential commodity, money. It's no coincidence that an industry with "overwhelming leverage" spends copious sums on lobbying. The Center for Responsive Politics reports that since 1998, the combined healthcare industries have spent $5.36 billion lobbying Washington. Compare that to the paltry $1.53 billion spent by defense and aerospace and $1.3 billion spent by oil and gas—two industries closely associated with lobbying.

On a personal note, working in a fee-for-service world created novel challenges like wondering how much is a reasonable charge for writing a prescription, listening to a heart, cleaning out ear wax, and listening to complaints (though there are set charges for specific CPT codes, as explained later in *Getting the Right Price*). In the U.K., doctors never have to sully their hands with money. They just get a salary or capitation per patient, regardless of what they do for each person.

The significance of this litany of ways the industry buys influence is that your best recourse is to become medically emancipated. But that goes beyond overseeing your medical care. To better help yourself, become politically active. Persuade your Congressional representatives that your displeasure is more of a threat to their political careers than the industry contributions are a help. Unfortunately, that poses a bit of a challenge.

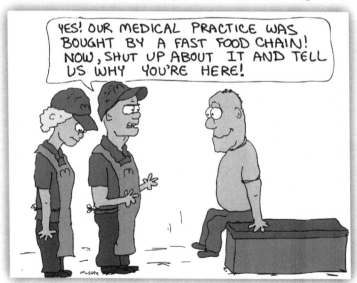

A FEW LOGISTICS

When talking about "doctors," I refer to regular allopathic doctors (M.D.s or D.O.s). In the term, I also include those collectively referred to by the rather unflattering title of "extenders," or nurse practitioners and physician assistants, who usually do as good (or better) a job as your primary doctor, but who are paid a lot less.

Those others who practice something besides good old respectable Western allopathic medicine are discussed in the Complementary and Alternative Medicine section (though the latest trend is referring to it as "complementary and integrative health) of *Getting the Right Treatment*. At the risk of sounding prejudiced—although I believe many do great work—they must be content to be called "therapists."

For the sake of brevity, I use the pronoun "he" for doctors, rather than "he or she" or the more politically correct "she." There are obviously many, many fine women doctors, and I don't mean to be sexist or exclusionary or belittling with my pronoun.

Doctors like to use *lingua medica*, those technical Latin terms. It sounds learned and exotic, even though it often turns out to be positively banal if you translate it (the big hole in the base of the skull, for example, is named just that: the *foramen magnum*). At the risk of deminishing the mystique, I keep this to a minimum for the sake of the laypeople.

Then there's insider lingo, as any profession has. Often, it captures black humor that can sound a bit derogatory, but it's a badge of membership, a spurious defense mechanism, or even a backhanded sign of affection. I use this lingo, but explain it, so you can feel like part of the club.

Of course, I also use the term "patient" a lot. To many, it has a somewhat condescending connotation. It's derived from the Latin verb *patior*, meaning "to suffer," or to be in pain or show forbearance. I use it, but it doesn't quite jibe with the empowerment I seek to facilitate with this guide.

But the alternatives thrown around these days, like "client," "consumer," or "resident" if the patient is housed in some institution, seem too cheesy. Sorry, if sticking with "patient" makes me sound like a conventional, paternalistic old bugger.

Finally, human beings are awkward creatures liable to have medical conditions manifest in their own individual ways. Every patient is different, and there's massive variability in the type and severity of each illness. In some respects, this makes it impossible to give one-size-fits-all advice.

There's a real need and desire for people to be more involved in managing their own healthcare. Robert Johnstone of the International Alliance of Patient Organizations notes that what still "needs to happen is for doctors to come down off their pedestal and for patients to get up off their knees."

This sentiment spurred me to write this guide.

Having surveyed the field of publications out there, I tried very hard to avoid some of the common deficiencies and to cover the essentials to make this a useful, relevant, understandable, interesting, and entertaining guide to your medical emancipation.

I hope you find it so.

CHAPTER 1

GETTING THE RIGHT DOCTOR

———

THE FIRST STEP

YOUR PROFESSIONAL HEALTHCARE BEGINS WITH getting the right doctor. He's sometimes likened to a lover or spouse, such is the degree of intimacy and trust you can develop, though without the sex to reconcile after arguments (hopefully). Or, he's sometimes likened to the conductor of an orchestra, coordinating the care of a host of different providers.

But how do you choose this spouse? This maestro?

That's what this chapter covers, along with how to find the right hospital, ER, and specialist. I also include discussions on different types of practice arrangements and how certain types of difficult patients can sour the relationship.

For our purposes, "doctor" refers to any kind of provider. The information applies whether you're looking for a Medicinæ Doctor (M.D.), Doctor of Osteopathy (D.O., who by the way, is virtually identically trained, just with a little manipulation thrown in), nurse practitioner, or physician assistant.

However, I focus on the primary care doctor. Your general practitioner (G.P.) is the one you see first, usually a family physician or internist, a gynecologist for women, or a pediatrician for kids. If you're not in the market for a primary care doctor, but are looking for a surgeon or specialist, the advice holds.

PRIMARY CARE FROM THE PRIMORDIAL OOZE

Medicine is an ever-evolving field, with doctors becoming ever more specialized. But now there's something of a renaissance taking us back to an appreciation for the primary care doctor.

Long ago, hospitals were established by religious organizations. Nuns and priests tended to the sick in a philanthropic way (in stark contrast to today's corporate healthcare). Illness was seen as a moral turpitude and treatment was intimately tied up with penance and punishment. There's still an element of this punitive outlook today, particularly when patients "do it to themselves," as with things like AIDS among drug users and those who fail to practice safe sex, complications from obesity, and lung diseases in smokers.

Then the Greeks introduced rationalism, the Arabs chemistry, and the Jews hygiene (of course). Science started to have influence in the sixteenth century.

Gradually, three basic subtypes evolved. The apothecaries, who primarily prepared herb and chemical potions as forerunners of pharmacologists; the physicians, who doctored; and those sophisticated barbers called surgeons. They competed for business and jockeyed for recognition and respectability.

The whole thing was a mess. There were nineteen licensing bodies in the U.K. in the nineteenth century. Then, in 1815, the British Parliament passed an act upholding the novel idea that each of these players should have to "evidence that he possessed some knowledge of his profession," and a certain amount of organization and rationality was imposed.

The training and degree of sophistication gradually improved. Doctors, like any evolving animals, started developing separate phyla and species—not with specific anatomical adaptations like extra long fingers for the gynecologist or proctologist—but with sub-specialties like sleep medicine, undersea and hyperbaric medicine, reproductive endocrinology/infertility, developmental behavioral pediatrics, neurodevelopmental disabilities, clinical informatics, and many other specialties you (and probably most doctors) are totally unfamiliar with.

Now, in what almost seems a retrograde step in this evolution, we appreciate the merits (versatility and cost effectiveness) of the primary care doctor, the generalist, the Jack-of-all-trades. Primary care is enjoying a renaissance.

Unfortunately, there's a tendency for med students to shun the unglamorous, fuddy-duddy life of primary care doctoring. They all want to become highly paid cardiac/orthopedic/brain surgeons, interventional radiologists, invasive cardiologists, or the like. Maybe it's because the avaricious bastards have an unreasonable desire to pay off their medical school loans and prosper.

In a gloomy comment, Mark McClellan, director of the Health Care Innovation and Value Initiative at the Engelberg Center for Health Care Reform at The Brookings Institution, predicts a shortage of 91,500 doctors by 2020. There are provisions in the ACA to promote primary care that will hopefully help, though.

A DOCTOR'S PERSONAL EVOLUTION

Each doctor must go through an individual evolution along the highly competitive career path from grade school to college to medical school to residency to fellowship (perhaps) to practice. The process has an unhealthy dehumanizing effect in my experience, with a strong prejudice that how much you know is the only worthwhile attribute for being a good doctor (the "knowledgism" of which I spoke in the *Introduction*). There's an emphasis on left-brain "detached objective neutrality," in the words of Daniel H. Pink in his thoughtful book *A Whole New Mind.*

My medical school training in England was not so different, with its de-emphasis on the humanistic side and glaring curriculum deficiencies, like diet and alternative medicines. I was first introduced to products of the American system in my two-year residency to get a U.S. license to practice.

Maybe the predominantly Jewish, highly competitive, New "Yoik" culture at SUNY, Stony Brook was a bad starting place for a wet-behind-the-ears, naive, dweeby, Englishman straight off the boat. The residents were full of themselves and overflowing with factoids and information, but they totally lacked common sense or a grasp of people and the world. Everyone's worth was judged by how much they knew.

It was the frantic, backbiting, competitive nightmare luridly described in Samuel Shem's cynical book *The House of God* (which everyone was reading at the time I was doing this residency). It's also well portrayed in the TV program *Scrubs*.

Things have changed a little, though. On the recommendation of the Institute of Medicine in 2008, the Accreditation Council for Graduate Medical Education, in their compassion, imposed limits on the torture to which residents can be subjected. It probably still wouldn't get approval from a French trade union, but residents now only have to work eighty hours a week, a maximum of sixteen hours in a row, and should have at least one day off.

Of course, residents tend to be left-brained and lack the depth of knowledge or acquired wisdom of a seasoned doctor, particularly when brand new. In July, medical students go through a magical transformation into newly minted residents and start looking after patients in the wards. Shem gives a good resident-eye-view of this phenomenon, which is seriously freaky. So, savvy patients try to avoid getting admitted to a teaching hospital in July.

You may also encounter residents in a teaching hospital-associated outpatient clinic. But, whether inpatient or outpatient, even if they appear hideously arrogant with feigned confidence to cover their insecurity and naivety, humor them and approach these skittish animals with kindness. You may be able to show how a medically emancipated patient likes to be treated. Get to them before they become set in their unfortunate, conventional ways.

Medical education needs to change, claims Pink. The "keys to the kingdom" need to be handed over from these rigid left-brainers. We need right-brain "creators and empathizers, pattern organizers and meaning makers."

Pink's slightly odd labels aside, the point was illustrated by actress Megan Cole, who so skillfully portrayed the emotional distress of a terminal cancer patient trying to wring some feelings out of her doctors in Margaret Edson's play, *Wit*.

It's sad that we need some antidote to the dehumanizing effects of medical school, but that's what Cole has been doing. She put together a sort of traveling circus, "The Craft of Empathy," and makes the rounds to various medical schools, cajoling a little humanity out of budding doctors. She teaches how to communicate empathy with body language and do the things normal empathetic people do instinctively. She teaches the touchy-feely techniques of active listening and how to affirm the patient's story (as a rudimentary form of this, we were told in residency to punctuate the patient's story by nodding and saying "aha" in an encouraging way).

Incidentally, nurse practitioners and physician assistants don't travel quite such a long and arduous educational road. N.P.s are nurses with a bachelor's degree, though the two we had at one stage in our office were as competent as any doctor, and far more personable. They developed a faithful following of patients who would see the doctor grudgingly if they absolutely had to. P.A.s are science undergraduates who go on to do two to three years of further training. And again we had some scarily well-informed P.A.s over the years.

As an aside, I'm amused at how the image of doctors in the media has undergone an evolution. Gone is loyal, understanding, emotionally connected, kindly Marcus Welby. Gone is dashing, debonair Dr. Kildare or Ben Casey. Gone is wicked but charming Hawkeye from *M.A.S.H.* Now we have obnoxious, sarcastic, irascible addict Gregory House and hateful Doc Martin, with their obliviousness to patients wanting human interaction and having feelings.

WHERE TO START LOOKING

There are many factors to consider regarding whom you'll trust with your healthcare. The first step is to compile a list of players to choose from.

Most people start by asking friends, family, and colleagues for recommendations. This can be a good tactic with people who know you, as they can often make a good match. But you may get more informed suggestions from people in the healthcare business, like nurses, pharmacists, and social workers.

Many hospitals have physician-finder services. Insurance companies have lists, but they often only include their own providers. Of course, depending on the specifics of your coverage, finding an in-network doctor may be important. A number of independent sites, like www.zocdoc.com (which I found very user friendly), www.vitals.com, and www.angieslist.com, are other good resources.

Your state's licensing board tells you about in-state doctors. Go to the Administrators in Medicine website of the National Organization for State Medical and Osteopathic Board Executives at www.docboard.org/aim. Or, the McMillan Law Firm provides addresses and links to state medical licensing bodies at www.floridamalpractice.com/linksotherstatebds.htm.

If you're old-school, physicians are listed in that big yellow phone number directory thing that gets dumped on your doorstep: the Yellow Pages.

You may live in a place where you have no choice. I once did a *locum tenens* in a one-horse/one-doctor town in Australia. Those patients don't have the luxury of saying "This guy's an asshole" and going to the competition.

No competition might sound great for the doctor, but not so much. It means being on-call 24/7, feeling like you can never get smashed, and keeping the ambulance crew informed of your whereabouts at all times (this was in the days before pagers or cell phones). I took a little trip to a beach a few miles up the coast and they had to send Wally, the local ambulance bloke, to come find me. I don't know how the permanent doctor survived it.

Plenty of websites, like the aforementioned Angie's List, post patient reviews of doctors, too. A few others include www.ratemds.com, www.healthgrades.com, and www.wellness.com. Or search for the name and location of the doctor you want to know about and you should easily find this information.

This is probably the most common way people check out doctors, but personal comments are highly subjective and often from patients who had an unusually good—or more often bad—experience that motivated the review. And sometimes reviews are fake, posted by the doctor's staff or paid writers.

If you didn't assemble your shortlist using the state licensing board's site, consult it to confirm the doctors you're considering are licensed and legit. The licensing body also usually tells you if a doctor has had any malpractice cases or claims made against him.

The website Bad Doctors In the News (www.baddoctorsinthenews.com) has links to emotive stories about a few wicked doctors behaving in sleazy ways. It's not comprehensive, but it does provide links to other sites with good advice on checking out doctors.

ASSESSING COMPETENCE (DOCTORS SHOULD KNOW STUFF)

Finding a doctor who knows enough to treat you competently is pretty important.

To maintain his license, a doctor has to get so many continuing medical education credits, and this ensures some degree of up-to-date knowledge. The doctor gets credits by attending conferences, reading medical journals, taking tests, etc.

It's not an infallible safeguard, though. I listen to Audio Digest recorded lectures and take the quiz, but they send you the answers before you have to submit your answer form. If you attend a conference, you get credits even if you sleep through every presentation.

Board certification, though voluntary, better indicates competence, legitimacy, and being current. That said, I'm the worst exam taker in the world, but I passed the Family Practice Boards doing nothing more than listening to Audio Digest in the car, which suggests the standards aren't particularly high.

You can check out someone's board status at the American Board of Medical Specialties at www.certificationmatters.org/is-your-doctor-board-certified/search-now.aspx, at the American Board of Physician Specialists at www.abpsus.org/public-inquiries, or at the Federation of State Medical Boards at www.fsmb.org.

Some claim doctors educated at a top college, medical school, or residency program must be highly competent. You can find this out from the licensing board, too, and most doctors publicize this information in their online bios and have certificates on the wall in prestigious-looking gold and black frames. Go to *U.S. News and World Report* at grad-schools.usnews.rankingsandreviews.com/best-graduate-schools/top-medical-schools to see how a doctor's institution ranks.

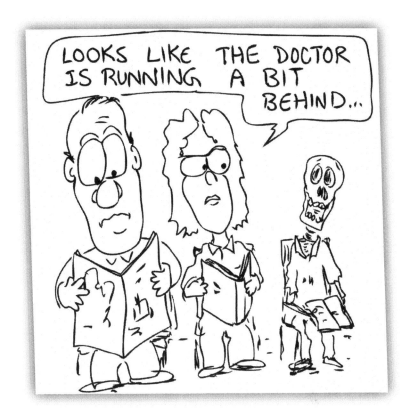

CONSIDERATIONS WHEN CHOOSING A DOCTOR

Consider whether you might be more comfortable with a male or female provider; many people prefer a doctor of the same sex, particularly when gender-specific issues arise. Female doctors reportedly spend more time with patients and may be more empathetic.

Age is a consideration, too. Older means more experience, probably from life as well as years in practic. Much of the advice I gave parents, like how to treat lice, diaper rash, colic, etc., came from having kids myself rather than from anything I learned in medical school or residency. But some old farts are more stuck in their ways, less adaptable, and perhaps less up on the latest and greatest. On the other hand, the young bucks may be oversold on the newest technologies and treatments and more likely to recommend drugs when lifestyle changes could suffice.

Punctuality is a hot-button issue and the leading complaint about doctors. Good doctors accumulate more patients and get overwhelmed. I had a *Broomhilda* cartoon up in the office with the patient saying to the nurse, "So all this waiting is because he's busy, which must mean he's a really good doctor, so it's for my own good, right?" The nurse replies, "No, it's because his golf cart broke."

Sometimes a doctor gets delayed by an emergency, and patients are unpredictable animals. Often, though, you're waiting simply because the office booked a totally unrealistic schedule to try and bang through as many patients as possible to get rich.

Aristotelis Belavilas of Las Vegas didn't accept the status quo. He sued his pain doctor for keeping him waiting. He didn't receive much sympathy from the local medical community. "The lawsuit was a sign of a society bent on suing over every little thing," railed Dr. Ed Kingsley, president of the Clark County Medical Society. He didn't get much from the court, either, which awarded him $250.

Then there are all those touchy-feely things like your doctor's social skills, emotional intelligence (his ability to read your feelings and empathize), compassion, flexibility, religious beliefs, and how much of that left-brain "detached objective neutrality" he gives off.

Some doctors are more stubborn or arrogant than others. My nephew Michael says he likes his chiropractor best of the various practitioners he goes to because, "He'll admit when he's wrong and look things up when he doesn't know."

Also, doctors, like all people, are not without prejudices. Some have prejudices against gays, certain ethnicities, drugs, alternative medicines, or drugs versus lifestyle modifications. When treating pain patients, there is a bias reported against women. A study published in *The Journal of Law, Medicine and Ethics* in 2001 found "women's pain reports are taken less seriously than men's, and women receive less aggressive treatment."

There are also doctors who, to a greater or lesser extent, don't "believe in" conditions like fibromyalgia, restless leg syndrome, vitamin D deficiency, chronic Lyme disease, premenstrual dysphoric disorder, chronic fatigue syndrome, oppositional defiant disorder, and even depression.

At the top of this list may be gluten sensitivity and celiac disease. "In medical school, celiac rarely gets the attention it deserves," laments The National Foundation for Celiac Awareness. There are doctors who "are either unfamiliar with modern diagnostic methods or unaware of the disease's true prevalence," it says.

If your doctor doesn't believe in what you suffer from, this could present a problem.

You may also need to consider what languages a doctor speaks, and certainly how effective a communicator he is. I'm reminded of when I was a flying doctor in Australia, seeing a string of pretty rough, tough stationhands on one property where we were doing a clinic (a table on the veranda). One guy told me, "Jeez, I'm crook, doc." Despite us both supposedly talking English, I had no idea what he was telling me. With a little effort, I ascertained that he was "feeling like crap," as it might be expressed in the U.S.

If a doctor doesnt' take the time or make the effort to express things in a way you can understand, this is no good. It's fairly common for doctors to lapse into jargon without realizing you don't know what they're talking about.

In her book *The Empowered Patient*, Elizabeth Cohen discusses seeing a doctor "with the communication skills of a potted plant." He was a surgeon, though, where it's possible communication skills aren't as crucial as other assets.

Speaking of potted plants, some people say not to go to a doctor if the plants in the office are dying.

Despite a lot of pissing and moaning about the problems of electronic health records, the general consensus is that they're good for patients. Their use should be a point in any doctor's favor.

Most patients prefer a doctor who shows them respect, which is something you have to feel out on an individual basis. One thing I always thought would put patients off is calling them by their first names, while the doctor expects to be called "Dr. So-and-So." But, in a survey reported in the *British Medical Journal* in 1990, out of 475 patients, 223 liked being addressed by their first names and 175 didn't mind. It was primarily patients over 65 that didn't like it. On the other hand, most patients don't want to call the doctor by his or her first name, the survey noted.

THE WHOLE PRACTICE MATTERS

It's not just the provider that needs inspection. When you become a patient, you take on the practice in its entirety, so you need to know things like whether the receptionist is a bitch and what the nurse is like; if the practice is anything like my office, the nurse is totally in charge of the doctor, and consequently worth schmoozing.

One colleague, a little on the wimpy side, had a nurse with a bunch of completely out-of-control kids at home. But she ruled him with an iron rod. I always joked that he was the only kid she could control.

More pragmatically, check out how long it takes to get an appointment and how easy it is to do so. Can you do it online?

What's the arrangement when your doctor's not in? Are his colleagues a bunch of jerks? What happens in the event of an after-hours emergency? How do you find out about lab results? Will the doctor give you advice by phone? Is he space age enough to communicate by e-mail?

TAKE THE DOC FOR A TEST DRIVE

To get a better idea, take a potential new doctor for a test drive, just as you would any car you were considering. He may be willing to do this as a free meet-and-greet. Otherwise, schedule an appointment to meet him or for some minor medical issue.

You might be permitted to accompany a friend or relative to an appointment if they're not going to discuss their impotence, hemorrhoids, or something else they don't want you poking your nose into. And, as long as the doctor doesn't feel you're tag-teaming him.

Feel out whether he's a good match. Pay attention to how punctual he is, whether he explains things clearly, whether he looks you in the eye or perpetually gazes at his computer, how he reacts to your out-of-control children, and his general appearance and personality. Check for horns and a tail.

It's better if you aren't shopping around for a new health-care provider during a crisis. If you're a procrastinator, you may suddenly be looking for a doctor when you're sick. That's not the best time to make a thoroughly researched, well-reasoned choice.

Within the profession, the cynical saying about the attributes that attract a patient to a doctor are, in descending order of importance: availability, affordability, affability, and last of all, ability.

FINDING THAT SPECIAL SPECIALIST

Looking for a specialist is a little different from selecting a primary care doctor. His licensing, disciplinary, and malpractice status are equally essential, but his personality may not be as much an issue. Surgeons are notorious for being a bit full of themselves. But maybe you can live with it if he's a gifted handyman. To me, though, nothing is more important in a surgeon—not even his dexterity—than his ability to make the right decision about whether you need surgery and if so, what type.

Usually, your doctor expects to choose the specialist you see, but the old-boy network often comes into play. You may get sent to someone simply because he refers patients to you doctor, because he's a drinking buddy, or most likely because he's a member of the same medical group or practice and your doctor wants to keep the business "in the family."

Your doctor tells you what specialist you need, but it isn't always as straightforward as it sounds. If a patient has a kidney problem, sometimes it's hard to decide between a nephrologist or a urologist, for example. A patient I saw recently with an apparent growth in her lungs and enlarged lymph nodes on a CT scan was a toss-up between a pulmonologist, a thoracic surgeon, and an oncologist.

With many types of cancer, it's a tough call between the specialist (usually a surgeon) who deals with that particular organ or area and an oncologist who deals with all cancers. If the patient needs surgery and chemo, sometimes both specialists are necessary.

HealthGrades (www.healthgrades.com) is a good resource for searching for different types of specialists by field, health condition, or treatment procedure. It also provides information about patient satisfaction rates.

The American College of Surgeons (www.facs.org) gives a lot of useful information on finding a surgeon under "Looking for a qualified surgeon?" Your decision should be based on outcomes, complication rates, and experience. I guess somebody has to be the first case, but better if it's not you. The more times someone's performed the operation the better.

If you're contemplating a prosthesis (a hip or knee replacement, for example) or some other implant, find out what the surgeon would use. Research its track record. The surgeon's choice might be influenced by financial ties to the manufacturer, so check that out as well.

The only way I know of to check on this is to ask, which might be a bit confrontational. I am not aware of any surgical device equivalent of ProPublica's service for finding out about whether doctors are getting kickbacks from drug companies. But more on all this in *Getting the Right Treatment*.

If you need an operation or procedure, consider the hospital or facility where the specialist operates. I'll get to selecting a hospital below, but in general, a good hospital has good people on staff.

One trick for tracking down leading specialists in a particular field, especially for some obscure or weird condition, is to see who's publishing research papers on the subject. Look online using Google Scholar and see who's doing the research. Any recurring name is likely to be a top specialist and a good person to see (though some researchers are academics who don't see patients).

There's an often-overlooked benefit to seeing a specialist at a research hospital: the doctor's payment system. That might not sound like it should matter, but it does.

Polly Murray, an artist and housewife from Lyme, Connecticut, is famous as the first person diagnosed with Lyme Disease. She wrote a book about it called *The Widening Circle*. She spent years visiting her primary care doctor and various specialists, beating up on them in her frustration because they couldn't figure out what was wrong with her. She felt like they gave her short shrift and were trying to blow her off. She finished up with Allen Steere, M.D., then associate professor of medicine at Yale, an archetypal teaching hospital.

She was enchanted. "He was understanding and unhurried in his approach," and "here was a doctor who was ready to listen," she crows.

While reading this, what immediately struck me was that Dr. Steere was a salaried doctor on staff at Yale. Murray's local internist and rheumatologist, whom she complains so bitterly about being too time pressured, were practicing "medicine by the yard." They got paid in the usual way—by how many patients they churn through in a day. This makes a huge difference in the willingness to listen to someone in detail and devoting a couple of hours to taking the history.

One last thought: when talking to your primary care doctor about a referral, a simple but savvy question to ask is, "Who would you go to?"

TYPES OF PRACTICES

Some marked changes are taking place in the ways doctors' offices are organized. Different models may not be available in all places, but you may have a preference that influences your choice of doctor.

The trend is moving away from the traditional Marcus Welby-style practice, where one or more doctors function as their own independent business as partners and owners.

Medicine is undergoing "incorporation," as large medical groups and hospitals set up their own practices or buy up and take over private practices. Physician ownership has been dropping by 2 percent every year for the last twenty-five years, so more practices are now owned by hospitals than by doctors, reports Steven Z. Kussin, M.D., author of *Doctor, Your Patient Will See You Now*. He notes the default option these days is "managed care Goliaths" with a new tier of managerial staff overseeing "disengaged, salaried physicians."

These practices tend to be run more as a business, often with strict productivity requirements. Doctors are liable to feel less personal involvement and responsibility, and maybe to put in a little less effort and caring.

Dr. Eric J. Cassell, clinical professor of internal medicine at Weill Medical College of Cornell University, reinforces this in *Doctoring: The Nature of Primary Care Medicine.* He says primary care doctors are becoming cogs in a machine and an "interchangeable commodity" in a marketplace of managed care.

One newer trend attracting a lot of business is the innovation of urgent care clinics. They are usually relatively fast and convenient, open evenings and weekends and requiring no appointment.

They're often set up by national corporations like Concentra and U.S. HealthWorks or local players (such as NextCare, Patient First, and PrimeCare in my area). These "doc-in-a-box" clinics are appearing on every street corner like fast food vendors. They provide semi-urgent care, often as a quicker, cheaper alternative to the ER, for acute but not life-threatening illnesses like the flu, urinary tract infections, sprains, small lacerations, and rashes.

However, these clinics usually aren't good for ongoing care, preventive care, or becoming that "medical friend of the family" that's such a key role for a primary care doctor. But they're siphoning off all those simple, short, lucrative office visits a doctor needs in his mix to be able to afford to continue to look after the little old ladies on twenty medicines.

Out of desperation and misery from the modern-day hustle a doctor has to be part of (to some extent), people are trying out new models of care.

CONCIERGE MEDICINE

Concierge medicine is a relatively new phenomenon that started in Seattle in the 1990s and now involves some 5,000 doctors nationwide.

The doctor has a "panel" of usually 300 to 400 patients (in contrast to the norm of thousands) who pay a yearly stipend in the $1,500 to $2,500 range. In return, they get more of his time and attention, can call him any time, get appointments within a day or so that are usually longer, and get more preventive care and an in-depth annual physical. There are often other perks, like the doctor coordinates specialists or sometimes even goes to the appointments with the patient, or accompanies him to the hospital.

This can be an appealing setup for doctors burning out on busy production-line medicine. They can make the same money seeing far fewer patients if they have receipts of $450,000 to $1,000,000 from the stipend, in addition to billing the patients' insurance. And the patients who can afford it love it.

Unfortunately, doctors usually drop a large chunk of their practice to do this. Our local paper reported on a Beverly Hills doctor who went from 2,000 to 400 patients; those 1,600 patients who won't or can't pay for an annual stipend were left in the lurch.

"Concierge medicine is not considered the ideal model for primary care medicine," says Glen Stream, M.D., board chair of The American Academy of Family Physicians. But he recognizes why physicians have made the switch as an "adaptation to a dysfunctional healthcare environment."

That's fairly mealy-mouthed, I'd say. Concierge medicine seems to me to create an obnoxious, discriminatory system that highlights the imbalance in care based on ability to pay. It dramatically reduces the country's primary care capacity, which is already suffering a serious shortfall as trainee doctors set their sights on more lucrative specialties.

MEDICAL HOMES

Other models affect how the doctor integrates with other members of the healthcare team, as with so-called medical homes, for example. They came about as a proposal of the American Academy of Family Physicians, American Academy of Pediatrics, American College of Physicians, and American Osteopathic Association to try to provide "accessible, accountable, comprehensive, integrated, patient-centered, safe, scientifically valid" care, according to a 2002 report, "The Future of Family Medicine."

Each patient has an individual doctor supported by a team of nurses, pharmacists, social workers, psychologists, nutritionists, physical therapists, and administrators who provide all components of care and 24-hour on-call coverage for urgencies.

The care is slightly less personal because you have several group members taking care of you. On the upside, different expert team members share common records, so care is much less fragmented; currently, the average 65 year old in the U.S. receives care from seven different disconnected providers, which is certainly not an ideal situation.

ACCOUNTABLE CARE ORGANIZATIONS

Accountable care organizations (ACOs) incorporate multiple practices, sometimes including multiple medical homes. They include specialists, hospitals, and all the same support staff as medical homes, working together in what have been dubbed "medical neighborhoods."

A key innovation of ACOs and medical homes is that they get paid according to patient outcome, not according to the traditional fee-for-service method. Any extra expenses come out of a central fund, reducing the doctors' profits. This provides financial incentive for good preventive care. One would hope provision of good care is incentive enough in itself, but let's not be naive.

The various providers are incentivized to pay attention to common-sense sort of things. For example, the pharmacist makes sure the patient has and knows about his prescriptions, the home health nurse makes sure the patients doesn't get bed sores, the dietician arranges Meals on Wheels to help maintain good nutrition, and the occupational therapist makes sure there aren't throw rugs for the patient to trip over. This keeps complications, hospital admissions, and other expensive interventions to a minimum.

The Affordable Care Act contains provisions that encourage ACOs and medical homes with the hope that they'll slow the runaway cost of healthcare. Some people worry it provides incentives to cut corners, and others say it's more likely patients only see a nurse practitioner or physician assistant rather than a real live doctor. But supporters counter that the incentives for more efficient, better integrated care far outweighs the drawbacks.

CHOOSING A HOSPITAL

If you need admitting or outpatient hospital services, you should pick a good hospital.

In an emergency, you often don't have a choice; the ambulance is generally obliged to take you to the nearest hospital. People tend to opt for the convenience and familiarity of their local hospital, especially if their doctor is on staff there. But convenience (and how much the hospital charges) does not correlate to survival, cautions Kussin.

Fifty percent of the time, people choose a hospital based solely on the recommendation of a friend. As with picking a specialist, though, if you have some more serious, obscure, or specialized problem, you may want to pay closer attention to hospital selection.

Hospitals tend to specialize these days. Memorial Sloan-Kettering and MD Anderson hospitals specialize in cancer treatment, for example, while Massachusetts General has a connective tissue clinic and Inova Mount Vernon Hospital has a joint replacement center.

If you need an operation, find a hospital that has performed it many times (as you want a surgeon who's performed it many times). High volume is good; the complications for bariatric surgery are twice as high (4 percent versus 2 percent) and the mortality rate for lung surgery is ten times higher in low-volume hospitals. Complication rates are a very important factor.

SAFETY

I always tell my patients—only half facetiously—that hospitals are dangerous places. Complications and medical errors in hospitals are a big issue these days, brought to everyone's attention by the Institute of Medicine's (IOM) November 1999 report "To Err is Human." It noted the number of people dying from medical errors is the equivalent of a fully loaded jumbo jet crashing every day, killing six times as many people as AIDS at the time. You'd probably expect it to generate a massive outcry, but somehow it's just seen as the cost of doing business in the healthcare field.

Some claim the IOM numbers markedly underestimate the danger. A report published in the September 2013 *Journal of Patient Safety* suggests overall there may be as many as 440,000 deaths per year from medical errors, making it the third leading cause of death in the country. Not all occur in hospitals, but some form of harm accompanies 25 percent of hospital admissions, according to cardiologist, geneticist, and author Eric Topol, M.D., who also notes that 42 percent of Americans report someone in the family has been the victim of medical errors.

This got people fired up to make some improvements, but results are hard to find. A study tracking 2,341 admissions conducted between 2002 and 2007 by ten respected North Carolina hospitals found no improvement in the rate of sixty injuries per

1,000 patients, despite all the outcry and implementation of systems meant to reduce medical errors.

There are major differences in risk between different hospitals. Kussin reports a possible threefold greater chance of dying in a casually chosen hospital bed than a researched choice. A little due diligence seems worth the effort.

The most common place for errors to occur is at admission or discharge. This is usually a problem of inadequate communication (responsible for 50 percent of medical errors), which is likely to be exacerbated if care is handed over to a different doctor because your own doctor is not looking after you in the hospital. In my experience, some medicine the patient was taking before admission or in the hospital often gets overlooked and not prescribed at discharge.

Look carefully at the hospitla's discharge medication list and compare it to what you were on before admission. Ask your doctor or the discharging doctor about any discrepancies. Also, check on any other discharge arrangements, like a home health nurse, physical therapy, and follow-up appointments.

If the hospital uses MAR (medication administrative records, which has all the details of your medicines), this reduces the risk of errors. Look for a hospital that uses this system, though not many do yet. Some self-empowerment advocates go so far as to tell you to insist on being given a copy of your MAR printout each day, though I have a feeling you would meet some reluctance.

Hospital-acquired infections are also a hot-button issue. A variety of bugs tend to colonize different "fomites" (objects capable of carrying infection) in the hospital. The claim is the TV remote is the most dangerous.

Twenty to 50 percent of patients in the hospital are colonized with one of the commonest contaminants, *C. difficile*, a pernicious bug that gets into your GI tract, especially if you've been given a lot of antibiotics, and causes a life-threatening gastroenteritis/diarrhea. But there are others, like the infamous MRSA. Kussin advocates taking your own hand sanitizer for the staff to use if you're admitted in case none is supplied, as well as posters to hang in your room demanding that everyone touching you wash or sanitize their hands first, which doctors in particular are so bad about doing.

Evidence-based protocols improve patient safety. A study of three hospitals in Michigan showed that using a checklist to ensure proper procedure and sterilization technique when placing a central venous catheter saved 1,800 lives over eighteen months. If you're having an invasive procedure, it's worth asking about the protocols and whether they're being followed.

Interestingly, smaller community hospitals often do better than bigger ones. In large urban hospitals, you're 15 percent more likely to get an infection (and likely to pay up to 30 percent more for the privilege), warns Kussin.

Look into the complication, infection, and mortality rates for any hospital you're considering for any procedure. The hospital should provide you with this information.

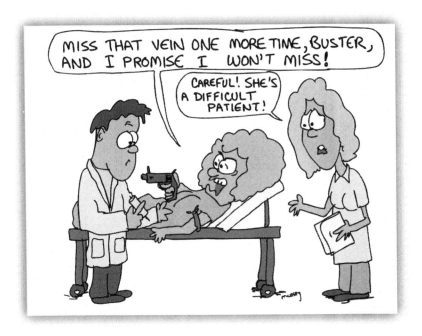

HOSPITALISTS

The trend gaining popularity since the late 1990s is for hospitalists, not primary care doctors, to look after patients in the hospital. Hospitalists are doctors who only look after inpatients at their hospital.

Hospitalist numbers have grown to about 30,000. Nowadays, only one-third of inpatients are seen by their primary care doctor. The Institute of Medicine says this is undesirable, as continuity is a defining attribute of successful primary care.

Some prefer hospitalists, but usually people prefer their own doctor who knows them. In the old days, when my group took care of patients in the hospital, it was nice to know exactly what had gone on with my patients. It can be tough on the doctor, though, as it's a bit like having two jobs, and I always seemed to be in the wrong place at the wrong time. When there was some crisis at the office, I was making rounds at the hospital. Or I was busy in the office when a patients was "crumping" (as it is expressed in the professional vernacular) and going down the tubes at the hospital.

Hospitalists have the advantage of being on site all the time and being more familiar with inpatient protocols, which can be a whole different world from office practice. So, when something goes wrong with a patient, or the insurance company suddenly denies further time as an inpatient, or there's some other urgency, someone is there to take care of it.

To bring up a rather delicate point, hospitalists tend to be foreign medical graduates. Of course, I myself am one, so I don't mean to sound prejudicial, but 25 percent of doctors in the U.S. are now FMGs, and in my experience they tend to be of a very left-brain, gung-ho, "do everything" mentality. This in contrast to your own low-key doctor who may be more willing to see how it goes, to use the "tincture of time," and generally be less aggressive.

If you don't want to be looked after by a hospitalist, keep this in mind when choosing a doctor and find one who attends at the hospital.

FINDING INFORMATION

Multiple organizations assess and rank hospitals to help you know where to go.

The equivalent of checking a doctor's license is to see if the hospital is accredited by The Joint Commission at www.joint-commission.org/accreditation/hospitals.aspx. Here you can also find out what specialized facilities a hospital has.

The Join Commission also accredits overseas hospitals. If you're traveling and want to know if there's a local hospital that doesn't use secondhand surgical gloves or rusty needles, check the site.

U.S. News and World Report is the best known private ranking organization, assessing hospitals since the early 1990s. Topol notes their ranking system is contentious because they go by "reputational score," which isn't reliable or objective because it's basically just a reflection of public image. It ranked the Cleveland Clinic top for geriatrics, even though the hospital has no geriatric department. It does however choose hospitals accepting the most challenging cases, which is significant because there's a tendency for hospitals to reject the tough cases, as they make their stats look bad.

HealthGrades (www.healthgrades.com) also assesses all hospitals. See how a hospital ranks for a bunch of different complications, like postoperative infections, hip fractures, or blood clots.

Kussin says www.WhyNotTheBest.org is the "absolute number one, hands down, thumbs up favorite," with a rigorous methodology and current statistics that allow you to compare hospitals for multiple different criteria.

Leapfrog (www.leapfroggroup.org), with the goal of supporting and promoting quality and transparency in healthcare for consumers, ranks 2,000 hospitals according to different metrics, like medication mishaps, appropriate ICU staffing, managing serious medical errors, and others.

Thomas Reuters ranks the top 100 hospitals by objective metrics, like risk-adjusted mortality, complications, re-admissions, length of stay, cost per discharge, and patient ratings.

It's confusing and a bit daunting trying to make sense of all these different agencies. There seems to be little consistency. Where one site ranks a hospital in their top ten, another doesn't even list it. This puts people off; only about 15 percent of patients use hospital scores to decide where to go.

The best advice I have is to look at several different sites and get a blended impression of any particular hospital. Though Topol comments that "It is essential, if at all possible, to have a go-to physician expert when one has a newly diagnosed, serious condition."

As noted, teaching hospitals usually have staff doctors at the top of their game and the most expert in their field. But again, they also have residents some people are not happy about.

Teaching and other large hospitals often have a suite for relatives to stay in, which may encourage you to go there. Also, take ancillary services like labs, radiology and imaging centers, outpatient surgery, physical therapy, and rehab into account.

Apparently, administrators think opulent-looking hospitals with chic furnishings and potted plants everywhere are good draws, given the fact that they're all built to look like five-star hotels these days. But don't get distracted; what really matters is a hospital's track record.

CHOOSING OUTPATIENT FACILITIES AND EMERGENCY ROOMS

As always, it's good to know where to go before a crisis hits.

Much of what makes an ER attractive are the capabilities of the parent hospital. Freestanding ERs with no parent hospital are a new phenomenon, but it's a considerable disadvantage that you have to be shipped off elsewhere if you need admitting.

Prefer an ER functioning out of a well-equipped hospital with features readily available on site like invasive radiology and radiologists, cardiac catheter capabilities, trauma management, cardiothoracic surgery, neurosurgery, vascular lab capabilities, and "clot busting" (fibrinolytic) treatment for heart attacks and strokes, when every minute counts.

To learn about the doctors staffing the ER, go to the American Board of Medical Specialties at www.abms.org.

Administrators also obviously think short ER wait times are a selling point, and it certainly might influence your choice. Nowadays, area hospitals become locked in pitched battles, displaying wait times in minutes on constantly updating electric billboards, like it's a stock market or racetrack odds.

Urgent care is a sort of halfway house between doctor office and ER. To know if one's up to snuff, look for the Certified Urgent Care designation from the Urgent Care Association of America.

MAINTAINING GOOD RELATIONS WITH YOUR DOCTOR

To go back to primary care doctors, in the interest of a harmonious relationship, I thought it useful to touch on some situations that challenge your doctor or might make him see you as a difficult patient.

There's plenty of folklore and medical literature about difficult patients, as well as some unkind nicknames some doctors have adopted, like "heart-sink" and "black-hole" patients.

Then there's *The Field Guide to the Difficult Patient Interview*, which makes it sound like doctors deal with wild and exotic animals (which may not be so far from the truth). It paints a morbid picture of a subset of patients who are hard to deal with. "Insistent or demanding of time and attention ... with overt or barely submerged anger."

You may think this is unfair and ask, "Where's the literature on the difficult doctor?"

Try Googling *difficult patient* and *difficult doctor* to get an idea of the profession's view of who's the difficult one. For difficult doctor, all I got was Dr. House, though some doctors probably agree with the his cynical line, "Treating illness is why we became doctors. Treating patients is actually what makes most doctors miserable."

Some categories of difficult patients are worth identifying.

Litigious Patients

Doctors are anxious about being sued for malpractice, so any patient that seems the slightest bit litigious may not receive a warm welcome. On average, a doctor is hit with a lawsuit every eight to ten years, regardless how careful he is. So doctors tend to adopt a not-if-but-when attitude.

Despite a lot of noise about needing to institute changes to reduce medical errors, as noted, there has been remarkably little progress. Errors occur, and it's not unreasonable that victims get compensated. But a lot of people think dealing with often complex issues in front of lay jurors, where some charismatic showman lawyer can hold sway and prompt awards of millions of dollars, is not a good system; rather, there should be tribunals with expert judges.

Malpractice premiums have passed their zenith, when brain surgeons and obstetricians in some states were paying yearly premiums around $200,000. Malpractice insurance companies hold seminars trying to reduce risk by persuading us doctors out of our bad habits, like losing vital test results in the mess on our desks and writing prescriptions in Sanskrit so the pharmacist can't tell if it says Celexa or Celebrex. But the cost of malpractice premiums and "cover your ass" (CYA) medicine, with its excessive testing, still adds significantly to the cost of healthcare.

Innovations at places like the University of Michigan Health System seek to reduce the litigation industry. UMHS is trying a new "humanistic approach."

If a mishap occurs, or if there's a complaint or a near miss, there is a full investigation involving the patient, family, and their attorney. An apology and reasonable and prompt compensation are offered if it's found the hospital made a mistake.

The problem with the present system is that by shutting down and refusing to talk for fear of providing the prosecuting attorney with ammunition, "we have given the patient no alternative but to sue," notes C. Boothman, Chief Risk Officer at UMHS. "And then we use the fact that they sue to show how opportunistic and awful they are," he said in a *New York Times* report on the results of the University's new policy for dealing with errors.

They say the best defense against getting sued is to be nice to patients, which can be difficult when confronted with some hateful person who, together with some ambulance-chasing lawyer, wants to nail you to the wall.

Hopefully it never gets to that for you. Just be aware, a generally better option is to discuss with your doctor why you are unhappy and try to enlist his help, rather than become his adversary.

NONCOMPLIANT PATIENTS
Few things on the patient's end jeopardize the relationship with the doctor like failing to do what he tells you.

This isn't just petulance or a feeling of being disrespected on the part of the doctor. Noncompliance accounts for up to 69 percent of all medication-related hospital admissions (costing $100 billion per year), up to 25 percent of hospital and nursing home admissions, and a threefold increase in doctor visits, according to Dr. Alan Showalter, writing on *Pharmforum* in April 2010. And there are the costs of morbidity in addition to monetary losses.

It's hard enough, even in our pill-obsessed society, to get people to take their medicines properly. The Office of the Inspector General tells us as many as 55 percent of elderly patients "do not follow medication regimens prescribed by their doctor."

If doctors could just get patients to comply with diet and exercise regimens, quitting smoking, drinking less, etc., there's no end to how much good we could do patients without medicine. Unfortunately, doctors are locked in an endless battle with the titans of industry selling cigarettes, booze, La-Z-Boys, and calorie-dense high fat/sugar/sodium foods.

Plus the pharmaceutical industry tries its best to keep the medical world so orientated to treatment with medications, endlessly encouraging that "screw the diet and exercise, I'll just pop a pill" attitude.

Compliance requires patient buy in. I find it helpful to simply tell people that this is what happens if they do this or don't do that, then they decide. More passive patients, like stereotypical little old ladies, tend to adopt the "whatever you think, dear, you're the doctor" attitude. But not everyone's like this.

Taking medicine several times a day is difficult, and medicines with their side effects can be scary. Fear of censure makes people hesitant to tell their doctor they're not doing what he told them to do. And it seems there's sometimes this perception that the the doctor's ego is tied up in patients liking the medicines prescribed.

When you take the doctor's advice and do what he says, it gives him the warm fuzzies, though also a tendency to take credit for the fact that you lost weight or quit smoking or whatever. But it is of course you that did the hard work and you that benefits.

There is one interesting new twist that will motivate your doctor to beat on you a bit more, though. These days, doctors are beginning to get paid by results, like receiving bonuses for the number of diabetics who have their hemoglobin A1c under 7.0 or hypertensives whose blood pressure is controlled. So, if you're some cussed noncompliant, out-of-control patient, you are not only tanking your doctor's stats, but you may be hitting him where it hurts most (hint: not the genitalia).

Obviously, compliance is important, so I encourage you to find a doctor whose advice you trust—and then take it. If you don't like what he's suggesting, see if you can negotiate some course that is acceptable to you both so you can still be compliant.

SEDUCTIVE PATIENTS

Seductive patients are also difficult. The stereotype is that the doctor is a dirty old man hitting on his vulnerable women patients, trying to get in their pants even when he's not doing a pelvic exam. But it goes both ways.

.

This obviously isn't a new problem, as there's a line in the Hippocratic Oath about prohibition of "all seduction and especially from the pleasures of love of women and men." The American Medical Association tells us we can't be romancing "concurrent with a physician-patient relationship."

Doctors are in a position to know some of the most sensitive and intimate details about a patient, making it the perfect job for a voyeur. The patient disclosing intimacies brings not just vulnerability, but closeness, and a bond that easily progresses into the patient feeling attraction toward the doctor. This is certainly exploitable by any lusty doctor.

I am intrigued to find this also works the other way around. It's called Florence Nightingale Syndrome, and I've even experienced it myself.

It's ironic that a syndrome having to do with romance/passion/lust is named after Florence, as she was a bit of a cold fish in that department. It's "Where a caregiver, typically a doctor or nurse, develops an emotional attachment to a vulnerable patient in his or her care." This may turn sexual, we are warned.

To make a very un-PC confession, I've found myself very sexually attracted to certain vulnerable, often depressed women patients. And certain patients use their sexuality to their advantage with the doctor, as some do in life in general.

One patient of mine was only in her early 20s, a hot ex-cheer-leader, on a pretty substantial dose of oxycodone for her "chronic pelvic pain syndrome," which always seemed to me a little sus-pect. But, she had been through the due diligence of going to the pain specialist and he condoned the treatment, so she came for her monthly visits to get her prescription.

She was always pushing the limits. She would want her pre-scription early for whatever reason, having taken more than she should have. She would want a little extra some months. She wouldn't want to have to pay for an office visit every month, so could she get a prescription for two months? And so on.

Bending any of these rules requires willingness on the part of the doctor. My wonderful, perceptive Bosnian nurse, Rasima, could see her doctor was putty in her hands.

Whenever she wanted some particular accommodation, her attire became noticeably more revealing and seductive. And "when she really want something bad," Rasima laughingly said to me in her Balkan English, "she will be absolutely naked!"

It's interesting that psychiatrists and psychologists, who don't go near or touch their patients, are particularly anxious about this sort of stuff. Actually, this anxiety is *why* they don't touch them. I had a job doing physical exams on new admissions at the local psychiatric hospital because of this aversion by the psychiatrists to laying hands on their patient.

Sometimes hormones override these honorable "hands off" scruples, judging by a Massachusetts report that 10 percent of psychiatrists admitted having sexual relations with patients. According to the psychological website www.kspope.com, a wicked 95 percent of male psychologists are attracted to their female patients. But maybe psychologists, not going through the emasculating experience of medical school, finish up a randier lot.

The rationale is that romantic relations between doctors and patients obscures objective judgment, and the medical disciplinary bodies take a hard line with professionals knocking their patients. The rules are even stricter for psychiatrists, as the American Psychiatric Association disallows sexual relationships with a patient even post-treatment.

There are accusations that the stiffs (if that's the right phrase in this context) on state disciplinary committees are just a bunch of killjoy, disciplinarian prudes. Isn't that always that type that seems to get onto those committees?

A case in Texas a few years ago saw an internist who began a consensual romantic relationship with one of his patients. He finished up in front of the state board, which imposed what some considered a swinging fine of $10,000, and he was required learn the error of his ways via ten hours of ethics education.

But, as critics pointed out, this same board dealt much more leniently with cases involving a feeding tube put into the wrong patient, an inadequate eye exam in someone with a traumatic eye injury, and a failure to meet the standard of care in a high-risk obstetric patient. All of these obviously had far greater potential to do harm.

Medically Emancipated Patients

Perverse though it may seem to include this section in my own book encouraging you to be a medically emancipated patient, sometimes such patients are considered difficult.

Some medical self-help books adopt a rather hectoring tone, telling their readers how to demand the doctor do their bidding, implying the doctor's some kind of foolish, reluctant animal that needs prodding along.

Sometimes it's not exactly appreciated when you bring piles of printouts of information you found on the internet and expect the doctor to read it all. Or when you run home after each office visit to look up what the doctor told you and call back demanding explanations why what the doctor said isn't exactly what WebMD says. Within reason, this may be good emancipated patient behavior, but it can be aggravating or threatening to your doctor.

Obviously, I am a believer in being informed and assertive, but try to be gentle and diplomatic.

Hypochondriacal Patients

Patients whose anxiety takes the form of constantly thinking themselves ill and wanting every little ache, pain, and apparent bodily malfunction investigated and explained can drive a doctor crazy.

We all have weird things happen to us from time to time. Some pain starts up for no apparent reason, but if ignored, it goes away. Doctors tend to develop an instinct for knowing what's a sinister symptom that needs investigating and what's not.

Much depends upon how wise and experienced you doctor is and how much faith you have in him. If he has a good track record, consider taking his word for it when he tells you don't need a brain scan, a blood test, or a referral.

PAIN PATIENTS

This is a double entendre, as patients being treated for pain often are a pain to the doctor.

It may sound unkind, but when treating people with narcotics—which is what all the most effective pain medicines are—there's always concern about the patient getting addicted or abusing the prescription. The potential prompts the DEA and other organizations to keep a watchful eye on us devious doctors.

We had a rather timorous, moralistic doctor in our office who refused to prescribe narcotics, so any patient with serious pain problems either didn't get treated or had to go elsewhere. This made me agree with Ben A. Rich, J.D., Ph.D., assistant professor of healthcare and law in Denver, when he wrote in the *Cambridge Quarterly of Healthcare Ethics* that you can't opt out of providing the only effective treatment for some people in the interest of "not being the subject of burdensome regulatory inquiry."

Prescribing narcotics, which are derivatives of morphine, which in turn is produced from those pretty opium poppies growing all over Afghanistan, always leaves the doctor concerned that the patient is faking or exaggerating the pain to get drugs. And, despite the fact that pain is now deemed the fifth vital sign, assessed by asking someone how much pain they have on a scale of 1 to 10, there's no objective way to know if someone's pain is really a 2 or a 5 or a 10.

The doctor must always be concerned about the potential for dependency. Is the patient taking it for the buzz more than the analgesic properties? Or, is the patient "diverting?" Oxycontin sells for about $1 per milligram. If you're on 80 mg Oxycontin twice per day, your month's supply has a street value of $4,800.

Other common prescription pain medicines, like Tylenol #3, Percocet, Lorcet, and Dilaudid, also have a significant street value. If you're some poor schmuck with a back problem eking out a living on disability, selling some or all of your medicine could be a bit of a temptation.

Prescribing pain medicine requires the doctor be a policeman as much as a doctor. It's a good practice to have patients sign a contract with strict rules about what they can and can't do (can't increase dose, can't get pain medicines from anyone else, must be willing to do a urine drug screen when asked, must be wiling to have prescriptions monitored through the state board, etc.). It's a major pain, and the DEA is always vigilantly monitoring doctors—and imprisoning not a few for over-prescribing.

The stereotypical image of the drug-abusing patient is some young hoodlum, but the two most egregious falsifications of scripts I have encountered were by little old ladies.

Most flagrant was Connie, with her fibromyalgia and arthritis. She would be brought to the office by her soft-spoken, dumpy, meek minister husband. He'd sit looking acutely embarrassed at the show she put on as she stridently complained about how her pain medicine was never enough, no matter how much I increased it.

After one visit, when I prescribed a small amount of extra Percocet for breakthrough pain, I got a call from the pharmacist querying about the script on which the twenty pills I'd prescribed had been deftly changed to 200.

If you require pain medicines, be aware of all this. Don't think your doctor's singling you out as a criminal because he wants you to sign a pain contract. Follow the rules; noncompliance with narcotics is one of the most common ways I know to get fired by your doctor.

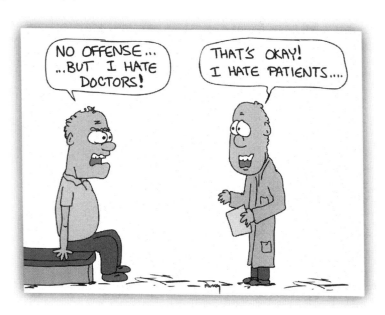

WHAT'S GOT YOUR DOC DOWN

Being a doctor is usually pretty well paid. It's also generally intellectually and emotionally stimulating and satisfying. It even commands a fair degree of respect, but there are lots of things about medical practice that can get your doctor down.

Understanding this may help you and your doctor have a more mutually respectful and rewarding relationship.

There's a massive amount of information for your poor doctor to know. On average, 39 percent of the day is spent doing busy work, according to Kussin. There are more and more regulations. There's financial anxiety, with 40 percent of medical students graduating with more than $200,000 of debt, while income and profit margins are constantly being shaved down. Doctors have to churn through so many patients every day to stay afloat (though "afloat" is a relative term, which some doctors consider inclusive of boat payments and country club dues). There's the constant threat of malpractice suits. There's the constant need for vigilance, lest there be some catastrophe buried in that humdrum parade of patients rotating through the office.

Dealing with sick and unhappy patients all day can be a downer, and especially emotionally exhausting when they are dying. Of course, it's particularly unpleasant being the harbinger of that bad news.

Doctors get burned out. As many as 40 percent suffer some degree of burnout, according to the AMA's September 2003 *Virtual Mentor*. They are likely to be "angry and irritable," and "Some become quiet, introverted, and isolated, which can be a manifestation of an underlying mood disorder. Others manifest burnout by over-eating or abusing alcohol or other mood altering substances. Still others experience chronic physical symptoms or diseases." Doctors contend with headaches, panic attacks, chest pains, muscle pains, and relatively high rates of divorce and suicide. There are reports of up to 27 percent of doctors being depressed.

Sounds like they need a doctor.

It can affect practice style and quality. The *Virtual Mentor* report notes other studies show that burned-out doctors have a bad attitude, make more mistakes, have a more expensive prac-tice style, order more procedures, and their patients are less compliant with prescriptions and follow-up appointments.

My experience is that cynicism is a common manifestation, often in the form of black humor, which also serves as a defense mechanism.

It certainly affects nurses, like when the ICU team was be-ing politically incorrect about a patient of mine and I put my foot in my mouth by writing about it.

I used to write *Dr. Gagg's Diary* for a local newspaper. One month I wrote about this patient who was small and already slightly funny looking. He had a leak from his lung that was forcing air out of his chest and under the skin, causing subcuta-neous emphysema.

This was causing massive puffiness. His cheeks were puffed out, his eyelids were swollen closed, his ears were enlarged, and even his scrotum was affected and looked like a water balloon. His skin had a funny crinkly feel, like bubble wrap, when you pressed on it.

Ever so discreetly and only amongst themselves, the nurses commented (correctly) that he looked like the nearsighted cartoon figure Mr. Magoo. As part of the team, I was privy to these bad jokes, and having the infallible judgment that I do, I wrote about it. Things weren't helped by the editor's tinkering, cutting out my delicately worded explanation of how this was the nurses' relief valve.

The powers-that-be at the hospital, which was of course always working hard on its image and promoting itself as an empathetic, caring "center of excellence," were not amused. They pulled the publication from the hospital and all the subsidiary facilities of their massive medical empire, which didn't exactly thrill the publisher.

FIRING YOUR DOCTOR

Sometimes a doctor pisses off a patient enough to make him want to find a new doctor. Some patient self-help books I've read talk about this like it's no big deal. But if you've been with your doctor for a while and he knows you and your family and maybe your whole medical history, it can be significant.

If you fire him, it puts you back in the market, dealing with the whole business of trying to find a new doctor you jibe with.

Far better than firing him is to have a frank talk to see if you can resolve the things about him or his practice that are driving you away. Even if this is difficult, it's often preferable to leaving and starting over.

Get your ducks in a row and make an appointment. You're much less likely to get good communication by phone or e-mail. Yes, you'll have to pay for an office visit, adding insult to injury, but it should be worth it in the long run.

When you confront your doctor, be specific about your problems, whether they're wait times, brusque office staff, poor follow-up on test results, difficulty getting appointments, condescending treatment by the doctor, or whatever.

Usually, patients simply move along to a new doctor without saying a word to the one they're leaving. The doctor just gets a request to send records on to some other office. This is less satisfactory for the patient and provides no opportunity for the doctor to learn something and perhaps improve things at his practice.

YOUR DOC'S PLACEBO EFFECT

Your doctor himself can act like a placebo. Just seeing him and getting a "dose of the doctor" can be therapeutic, even if no specific treatment is provided. This is a very helpful strategy for demanding patients with rather nebulous conditions or one there isn't much to do for, like bad arthritis, fibromyalgia, multiple sclerosis, cancer, emphysema, or some psychiatric conditions. It provides reassurance that the doctor is not abandoning the patient and is keeping an eye on things.

The longer you've been with your doctor and the better he knows you, the greater this placebo effect is likely to be. This is another good reason for not firing your doctor in an offhand way.

CHAPTER 2

GETTING THE RIGHT DIAGNOSIS

———

SO MANY STORIES

WOULD YOU LIKE TO HEAR about the guy from my local Unitarian church who was very short of breath with pains in his chest who—despite relating that he also had leg pains and a family history of blood clots—was given two rounds of antibiotics by the ER doctor who vehemently adhered to a diagnosis of pneumonia following a cold?

Later, he went for his flight physical and could hardly walk to the exam room. In desperation, he asked for the advice of the flight surgeon. It was only then he was sent for the CT scan that showed the pulmonary embolus causing the problem.

Or...

A patient of mine, Mary, was dragging, depressed, overweight, and her hair was falling out. She was told, "it can't be your thyroid because your TSH test is normal." She scoured the countryside and found a slightly offbeat gynecologist who cured her by putting her on an old-fashioned thyroid medicine.

Or...

My nephew, Michael, had intractable stomach symptoms blown off by multiple gastroenterologists as irritable bowel syndrome. They were cured when, on the recommendation of a friend, he went to a "Lyme literate" doctor (one of those controversial doctors who believes in the idea of chronic Lyme Disease) who cured him by testing and treating for an intestinal yeast infection and taking him off wheat products.

Or...

Trisha Torrey, speaker, author, and founder of health advocate website AdvoConnection, was diagnosed with the most aggressive lymphoma and was on the brink of having some particularly poisonous chemotherapy. Then she did her own research and figured out she only had inflamed fat cells (prompting the book *You Bet Your Life!: The 10 Mistakes Every Patient Makes*).

Or...

Jerome Groopman, M.D., wrote in *How Doctors Think* about the years of debilitating pain and swelling in his wrist. He consulted the best hand surgeons and, despite being a doctor himself, experienced that classic hurried, dismissive arrogance so many patients complain about. He had the confidence to reject the obscure diagnosis and surgery being pushed and kept trying till he found a doctor who made a diagnosis where everything added up. The history, the exam, and the X-ray findings all jibed and the relevent treatment finally got him better.

Or...

Polly Murray, a New England artist, spent years beating on the medical profession about her constellation of weird and wonderful symptoms that were repeatedly blown off as psychosomatic. Finally, she made so much fuss that Harvard Medical School took an interest in her case and Lyme Disease was discovered.

Everyone has a story about how they or a friend or family member were misdiagnosed or mistreated.

"Different surveys suggest that as many as 40 percent of all diagnoses are wrong," corroborates Michael Roizen, M.D. of the Cleveland Clinic and Mehmet Oz, M.D. of *The Dr. Oz Show* fame, in their book *YOU: The Smart Patient: an Insider's Handbook for Getting the Best Treatment.*

And you find yourself asking, "how can doctors be so stupid?"

It is, of course, easy to be wise after the event, with the "retrospectoscope," as the wags of medicine talk about. From a doctor's point of view, a lot of people have problems that are difficult to diagnose, some of which never get solved. It's not stupidity, but that the practice (a word to clue you in that this is not a definitive science) of medicine can be pretty damn tricky.

A common theme amongst people who get the most from the medical profession is they actively participate in their healthcare. They work with—rather than rely wholly on—their doctor.

THE FIRST ENCOUNTER

The process of getting the right diagnosis starts with "the encounter." Sounds a little hostile, doesn't it? But it's the first step toward your doctor arriving at the right diagnosis.

Every new primary care patient begins as a mystery, and the first encounter makes primary care a little exciting. Doctors never know what pathology or crisis lurks behind the exam room door. It's a bit like *Deal or No Deal*, telling Howie to open the case.

Despite the seemingly chaotic nature of the office (assuming your doctor's office is like mine was), the process follows a pattern: the so-called "SOAP note" format. That's not to suggest life in the office is an ongoing episodic drama (although it is); it's merely a way of dividing up the entire process. There's the Subjective, Objective, Assessment, and Plan. This makes everything easier to record. More on this in a moment.

PREPARING FOR THE APPOINTMENT

To get the most out of your encounter, be prepared (and be on time, just in case your doctor is). Make a list of what you want to address with the doctor.

This helps avoid the "by the way" issues doctors complain about so much. These are concerns the patient brings up at the end of the visit as the doctor impatiently stands poised to exit, hand on the door handle, when the patient finally tells him the real reason for the visit.

Give serious thought to what you definitely want to talk to the doctor about and what questions you have. It's not unreasonable to write down what you want to cover, but a smart doctor will ask to see your list at the start, so show it to him first and he can help prioritize it.

Bring as detailed a record of your symptoms as possible, and try to organize them chronologically. And please, supply your doctor with symptoms, not a diagnosis. If you complain of "ulcer pain" and the doctor takes you at face value, the Pepcid or Prilosec he prescribes won't do a bit of good for gallbladder pain, which has a cussed habit of producing pain very like that coming from an ulcer. Just just tell your doctor what you experience and observe and let him draw the conclusions.

When writing out your plans for the encounter, be realistic. I had one patient bring me a drawing using a stick figure to illustrate all the different parts and problems she wanted to cover. It was adorable, but it was a fifteen-minute appointment and there were fifteen bullet points.

The "laundry list" is a piece of medical folklore doctors joke and gripe about. If you turn up with a really long list, your doctor is liable to balk. You can't realistically expect thorough review of too many issues, so recognize that you may need more than one visit if, when you're jotting down your list, it begins to look like the Dead Sea Scrolls.

Along with your list of topics of conversation and symptoms, bring as much information as you can.

Put together your family history, including any quirks in the family tree that might be hereditary. Things like vascular/heart disease, diabetes, cancers, dementia, and mental illness have genetic components. Anything may be relevant, and the closer the relative affected, the more important it is. The ethnic makeup of your family can be important (certain illnesses occur disproportionately in certain ethnic groups), as can the place and environment where you grew up.

It's a common misconception that your doctor has access to all your tests and records. The more you bring, the better. One potentially helpful item is an old ECG, especially for comparison if you need another one; knowing whether any peculiarities were there before is incredibly helpful.

Inquire ahead whether you'll need to fill out any medical history forms, and ask if you can have them sent to you before your appointment. You can be more thorough if you're not trying to rush through them at the office.

Also, bring the original containers of all the medicines you take. The label has all sorts of information people often don't know offhand, like the date dispensed, who prescribed it, how many refills are left, and how it should be taken.

As a side note, if there's a language barrier between you and your doctor, you might try LanguageLine Solutions (www.languageline.com).

Armed with your list and information, you're ready for your starring role in...

THE "SOAP" OPERA

S Is For Subjective

This refers to your medical history. The nurse usually starts and the doctor delves deeper. Both want to know your symptoms, how bad they are, when they started, what makes them worse, and so on.

It will help—at least in your relations with your time-pressured doctor—if you are concise.

We're taught in medical school to pose open-ended questions, like "How are things going?" rather than leading questions, like "Do you have to get up at night to urinate?" But this lets patients take the lead and wander where they will. "It's going pretty well, but I had this pain when I went to visit my brother, you know, the one in Philadelphia who just bought a vintage Mustang. He threw his back out, and we were going out to eat, and there's a really good seafood restaurant there, right down by the river, I think it's called..."

We're also taught not to grab patients by the lapels and shake them, screaming, "Get to the point!" But this might have something to do with our reputation for interrupting patients within nanoseconds. And it's a fair reputation.

In a study published in the November 10, 1984 *Annals of Internal Medicine* by H.B. Beckman and R.M Frankel, only 23 percent of patients were permitted by their doctor to complete their initial statement about their agenda for the appointment; on average, doctors interrupted in eighteen seconds.

In reality, I always found it to be an ongoing to-and-fro, interrupting repeatedly but briefly, clarifying points as the narrative unfolds. There's a maxim from that wise old physician, William Osler, known for his aphorisms, that goes, "listen to your patient; he is telling you the diagnosis."

"Listen" is the operative word. I'm sorry to say, sometimes my colleagues are not the best listeners. But they do hear, particularly what is bugging you and what you think is important, even if it's not necessarily what he thinks matters.

In a feisty defense of doctors apparently not listening, "The Unhappy Hospitalist" tells us on his "unfiltered blog" that 90 percent of what patients tell doctors "is garbage," or at least doesn't provide useful information for a diagnosis or choosing treatment. And, as *The Field Guide to The Difficult Patient Interview* points out, doctors have little time to "ascertain the symptoms, make a diagnosis, get to know the patient in a broader psychosocial context, develop a therapeutic relationship, and counsel the patient about behaviors and therapies." And I would add: order tests, fill out any one of a zillion different forms, and write prescriptions.

Making a diagnosis is largely a computer-like function. Doctors mull over the symptoms and try to figure out which illnesses could cause them, like Sherlock Holmes pondering the clues to a crime. And, often, there's great satisfaction upon solving the mystery.

To do this, doctors need the facts to compute. The more precise those facts and the sooner they come to light, the faster and more accurately your doctor's churning computer-brain spits out an answer. A carefully taken history is the most important factor in making a diagnosis, much more so than any records or examinations or tests. The lament today, unfortunately, is that taking a good history is a dying art.

O Is For Objective

This is the physical examination... all that looking, prodding, poking (palpating), and using that irrefutable badge of the profession—the stethoscope—for listening to (auscultating) the many different parts.

Jessica is a lively but slightly bashful young physician assistant I mentored in the office. One day, she was presenting the case of a guy she thought might have an inguinal hernia (a rupture). In bad cases, a loop of bowel can push down through the inguinal canal into the scrotum.

One joy of teaching is when students come up with new ideas. Jessica broadened my horizons about the use of the stethoscope when she told me, "I auscultated his scrotum, but I didn't hear any bowel sounds." At least it's not like the old days, before

Laennec invented the stethoscope, when we had to press our ear to the part we wanted to listen to.

To facilitate your exam, wear clothing that's easily loosened, removed, and thrown back on when you have to sit around for hours in some diaphanous paper gown feeling cold and vulnerable. I once participated in one of those mass school gymnasium sports physicals and was allocated to the girl's side; the fashion for camisoles was a veritable nightmare.

Another plea: wear clean clothes and take a shower. I'm sure *you* always smell like a rose, but not everyone does. As a doctor who's sat on that little stool doing a pelvic exam, nose effectively buried in someone's crotch, I assure you, cleanliness really is next to godliness.

A Is For Assessment And P Is For Plan

Sometimes, the A and P are no-brainers. Maybe some woman who just got laid for the first time woke up the next day feeling like she had to pee all the time and the urine shows some blood and a bunch of bacteria. It's a pretty sure bet she has a bladder infection (or "honeymoon cystitis," as it's sometimes called, since women have intercourse for the first time on the honeymoon). She needs a short course of antibiotics.

Sometimes, a guy just needs the burn from the muffler on his motorcycle dressed. Sometimes, it's poison ivy.

We should always be so lucky. Often, the patient has pains, fatigue, weight gain, tingling, headaches, depression, bloating, insomnia, palpitations, dizziness, and every other nebulous symptom caused by any one of a zillion diseases. Such a patient is a serious WTF.

Part of such an assessment is compiling a "differential diagnosis," or a list of all the things that could be indicated by the symptoms. You'd think a computer would be ideally suited to this task, and there are such programs, but they tend to come up with very long lists that call upon all the small print esoterica. Computers aren't good at doing what doctors do, almost subliminally: singling out the more probable causes, keeping with that profound medical maxim, "common things occur commonly."

WHY YOUR DOC MAY GET THE DIAGNOSIS WRONG

There are pitfalls, and plenty of reasons your doctor might not figure out the right diagnosis. He may not get sufficient details out of you, like to differentiate between heart pain or stomach pain. Or, he may not go through your differential in a methodical way. The symptoms may not yet be telling enough; many illnesses, like diabetes, kidney disease, and high blood pressure, show little in the way of symptoms in early stages.

Or, maybe you have something he just never thought of. Pulmonary embolus and dissecting aneurysm of the aorta are two good examples of problems often overlooked in the differential.

There are also a lot of quirks in the way doctors' minds work. We are more likely to diagnose what we see a lot of. My smart-ass comment to everyone coming to my office in Virginia with a runny nose is, "this is the most allergic place in the world." I would immediately diagnose them all as having allergies, because allergies are so common where I live. But of course your runny nose may be a cold, overuse of nasal steroids, vasomotor rhinitis, a reaction to using cocaine, a leak of cerebrospinal fluid from an injury (hopefully not), and, if you look hard enough, lots of other obscure causes.

A doctor may be more inclined to diagnose something he was burned by in the past. When I was a "Houseman" (as they call junior hospital doctors in England) at an orthopedics firm, the nurse called one night to tell me a patient scheduled for surgery the next morning was having indigestion. I told her to give him some antacids (with a "stop bugging me!" subtext). Well, it wasn't indigestion; the guy was having a heart attack. For a long while after that, I diagnosed anyone presenting with "indigestion" or any kind of chest pain with angina and really put them through the wringer.

If it's an old patient or one coming from another doctor, a diagnosis has likely been made already and it's often just accepted without much thought. Being disciplined enough to constantly consider the pros and cons of each diagnosis is time-consuming, hard work, but good doctors keep an open mind. And they are not usually the ones getting the complaints.

To delve deeper into the quirks of the contorted mind of the doctor to better understand how they screw up, let's talk about "anchoring." A busy doctor, when confronted with some diagnostic challenge, often jumps to a conclusion and becomes immovable from it. At these times, the doctor may rationalize away or ignore evidence that doesn't fit the diagnosis with so-called "confirmation bias" or "diagnostic momentum."

This seemed to happen to Jerome Groopman, with his painful wrist problem mentioned earlier. He was first diagnosed with "overactive synovium," which he had never heard of. Then, it was pseudogout, which is very rare, so he was skeptical. The first two surgeons ignored clues that didn't fit with these diagnoses. The last surgeon's explanation seemed to add up; the diagnosis, the physical findings, the X-rays, and the MRI all pointed to the same thing, so Groopman had a gut feeling this was the correct diagnosis.

Many poor, insecure doctors, despite their air of aplomb and confidence, are afraid they look bad if they don't appear to know with certainty what is wrong. This too can prompt a jump to a conclusion and immovability. As Dr. Groopman notes, doctors feel a need to "behave with poise and an aura of competence, with denial of uncertainty, in front of patients."

This is all compounded by the doctor always being rushed, which makes hurried decisiveness a necessity. Presenting a host of possibilities and having to mull them over with the patient and answer all the questions this can prompt is the last thing a busy doctor wants to do, even though this is what makes the patient happy.

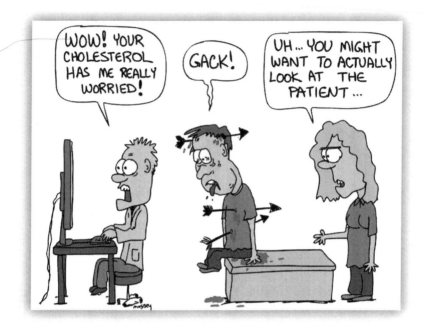

TESTING, TESTING, TESTING

The differential diagnosis must be whittled down. This often involves some kind of lab testing or imaging. However, some things, like skin conditions and psychiatric illness, don't have much in the way of helpful lab work, so the diagnosis depends on what in this day and age is often considered medical voodoo: the clinical acumen of the doctor. If your doctor is stymied by one of these conditions, you may go to a specialist for a second opinion.

Which tests to order (and how many) can really tax the doctor's judgment. All tests have down sides. They're inconvenient, expensive, painful, or dangerous. Plus, they're a pain in the ass and potentially costly for the doctor, too, when he needs one of his highly paid staffers to plead with the insurance company to get big ticket items like MRIs or nuclear stress tests or PET scans authorized. This preauthorization process can take a long time, too.

The insurance company's say in whether or not you can have a test (or, to be more exact, whether they will pay for it) is a contentious business that ruffles feathers when one of the carrier's bean-counters says no. The obvious criticism is that the insurance company's only concern is the cost, not getting to the right diagnosis. They favor doctors who order fewer tests.

Cigna and other insurance companies recently settled with New York State over accusations they were making lists of preferred providers for patients based on the amount of money the doctors saved the company. The system was "rewarding them for not rendering, in some cases, the best and most effective medical treatment possible," writes Richard S. Klein, M.D., in *Surviving Your Doctor.*

You may think knowing what tests are needed is a pure science, but "Medical necessity is a very subjective affair," says Steven Kussin, M.D., in *Doctor, Your Patient Will See You Now.* There are lots of reasons your doctor may be a bit overzealous.

In this information age, one of the more absurd reasons for doing lots of tests is that often your doctor just doesn't have the results of previous tests, so he orders them again. This particularly applies when you go to a specialist. Make sure all records get to your doctor, either by taking them with you or calling a few days beforehand to confirm they are there.

Your doctor may also be worried about missing something and getting sued, so he orders more tests. As a doctor, there's always the specter of some lawyer breathing down your neck.

I think ER doctors take the biscuit here, with their belief they have just one shot at a patient. A primary care physician or specialist tells his own patients to come back if it doesn't get better. ER doctors are prone to thinking that if they don't do every test, they'll miss something and the patient will sue them or die or both.

Sometimes your doctor—especially if he's a specialist offering a second opinion—feels compelled to order tests to justify his existence, to make you feel like he's doing something. If he doesn't come up with a different diagnosis or request more tests, and basically says he has nothing to add, you'll probably wonder, "Why am I wasting my time and money on this turkey?"

As I said, many factors prompt your doctor to order a bunch of tests. Since this is a key part of high medical bills, I discuss it more in *Getting the Right Price.*

DAMN LIES AND STATISTICS

Every test has statistics that indicate its usefulness. No test is perfect, any one can miss an abnormality (a false negative) or indicate an abnormality when there's not one (a false positive).

The "sensitivity" of a test refers to the percentage of true versus false negatives it detects. Mammography, for example, has a sensitivity somewhere around 95 percent in good hands; it detects up to 95 percent of breast cancers and misses 5 percent.

"Specificity" indicates the proportion of true versus false positives. Mammography has a specificity of approximately 97 percent. That means 97 percent of what is identified as a breast cancer is one, while 3 percent of what appears to be a breast cancer is not.

Needless to say, it's not good to have a false negative and tell a woman she doesn't have breast cancer when she does, as she will go untreated. Nor is it any good to have a false positive and put a woman through needless anxiety at the least, and possibly further testing or unnecessary treatments—possibly including some gung-ho surgeon pointlessly cutting her open.

As an important aside, the quality of the test and the lab and professionals doing it also affects any test's ability to rule a problem in or out (accreditation of labs is by various bodies, but mainly the Joint Commission and the College of American Pathologists).

The likelihood of a true positive versus a false positive is also affected by the prevalence of the disease in the community. For example, a positive blood test for the stomach bacteria *Helicobacter pylori* (which causes ulcer-type symptoms) is much more likely to be a false positive in a developed Western country where the incidence of *H. pylori* is low than in a Third World country where it's high.

A slight variation on false positives is that tests—especially imaging studies—often turn up some incidental finding that is pathologically insignificant but leads to further intervention. A review of 1,426 CT scans by the Mayo Clinic found incidental findings in 40 percent of cases, so it's not uncommon.

CT scans are a particular problem because the radiologist has an awful lot of pictures to look through. Yes, computers help by doing a pre-screen and highlighting any dodgy images, but still it's difficult. Plus, radiologists are cautious animals and tend to err on the side of caution to cover their backsides (Kussin accuses most X-ray interpretations of being "hedging, quasi-legal documentation").

This business of incidental findings can lead to real quagmires.

I had this patient, C.O. She was petite, pretty, in her late thirties, demurely dressed, with a hesitant and insecure manner and an air of vulnerability (which, as mentioned, I find a bit of a turn on, and that may be why I tolerated her foibles more than I might have in other patients). She was a "homemaker" whose husband was away a lot and whose 7-year-old son was having problems at school.

She was always listless and presented with nebulous symptoms like fatigue, dizziness, bloating, nausea, and anxiety, and she was especially worried about feelings of numbness in her hands and the side of her face. She told me her girlfriend had just been diagnosed with multiple sclerosis.

We started with a CT scan of her head for the dizziness, which came back showing "no definite cause for dizziness, but questionable abnormalities in the white matter," with the comment that "an MRI scan would help to clarify these."

So we proceed to an MRI scan. This came back saying, "some areas of high signal abnormal white matter on the T-2 weighted images which could be consistent with demyelination" (the *sine qua non* of MS). And, "this is probably normal, but repeat MRI with Gadolinium contrast would show these lesions better." Also, "the pituitary gland seems just above the upper limit of normal size."

Now, not only do we have findings that could be indicative of MS and require another test to be sure, but there's a question of whether there's something wrong with her pituitary gland, and maybe that has something to do with all her weird symptoms. Does she need an endocrine work up? Should we do a second MRI scan with contrast? All this in someone I'm convinced has symptoms that stem from stress and somatoform disorder because she seems such a classic case and doesn't have any other symptoms of MS, or of endocrine failure for that matter.

What do I tell her? "There's some possible plaque in your white matter and a possible abnormality of your pituitary gland, but I don't think we need to persue this further." That's one possibility I'm sure would go over well.

Or, I could trust my own judgment, adopt my best paternalistic style, and tell her "there's nothing we need to worry about here." Then what do you suppose this rather hypochondriacal patient's reaction would be if she sees the report?

Maybe you're thinking it sounds positively negligent not to pursue abnormalities like these. This whole hurdy-gurdy went on for years, with all different tests showing questionable abnormalities but never coming up with anything definitive. C.O. never got worse, nor did she die. But telling her "We've done so many tests, I think it's highly unlikely you have some physical disease we haven't discovered yet" wasn't going to cut it.

With any test, the "normal" range is a bit arbitrary. The numbers we pick as normal or desirable aren't set in stone, but are decided by some expert(s). The recommended goals for total and bad (LDL) cholesterol keep getting revised downward, for example, not to mention the recommended tests keep changing, too. Total cholesterol is "so 90s," complains Kussin, who says you have to look at cholesterol sub-particles these days.

A "normal" range is simply where 95 percent of the population falls, and any reading outside it is "abnormal." It's possible to be outside the normal range and be fine, though it's less probable.

Tests as basic as blood pressure readings, which are generally done on every patient at every visit, should be subject to the same disciplined approach involving assessment of the pros and cons as more elaborate (and costly) tests. It is my opinion that many doctors overreact to elevated readings and put people on blood pressure medicines, or even ship patients off to the ER, without adequate justification.

I have some support from the Joint National Committee, which recently revised the guidelines for treating hypertension (published in the *Journal of the American Medical Association*, February 2014), recommending slightly less stringent criteria.

Also, there's no point doing a test if you can't do anything with the result. If it uncovers some condition for which there's no cure or effective management, what's gained by knowing?

Considering the pros and cons of tests is particularly important with screenings like mammograms, PSAs, colonoscopies, and cardiac stress tests, especially when ordered for people with no relevant symptoms. Strict criteria are in place for what makes a screening test valid. The benefits have to outweigh the downsides. Downsides include the results of a false positive or incidental finding of something that isn't going to do you any harm, as well as potential dangers of the test itself.

Overuse of mammography may cause cancer by exposing women to radiation. It's not very much, but it's estimated that approximately 2 percent of all cancers in the U.S. may be related to ionizing radiation such as that from X-rays. CT scans provide much more exposure, and enthusiastic American doctors do about twice as many CT scans per capita than those in other countries (20 to 40 percent of which are claimed to be medically unnecessary).

Some prey upon the public's lack of awareness about the downsides to screenings. Companies like HealthFair and Life Line Screening park their "scan-in-a-van" outfits at churches, hotels, and malls, playing on peoples hypochondriacal tendencies with glitzy brochures proclaiming "Tandi Clubb can shout

'I owe my life to Life Line Screening'" because she was found to have some atheroma buildup in her carotid artery.

They neglect to mention the further tests and anxiety created when their scans identify incidental findings and false positives. They also fail to disclose that the government organization that carefully analyzes the validity of tests, the U.S. Preventive Services Task Force, does not recommend using the tests these companies offer for screenings (as opposed to using them for further information about a known pathology or to diagnose observed symptoms).

Perhaps I have a bee in my bonnet about unnecessary screenings, since I recently allowed myself to get suckered into what I would guess was a not-very-worthwhile test at my dentist's office.

I have Medicare, and dentistry isn't covered (please, someone tell me why not), so I was a "self-pay."

I thought I was just going for a checkup, but was immediately assailed by the hygienist. All the poking and scraping was bad enough, but then she declared, "You haven't had a panoramic X-ray in a very long time." And shaazzaam, I'm standing with my head in this sort of helmet X-ray machine attached to the wall and my bill is $220 instead of $35.

I seriously question whether the X-ray was necessary. What's more, though, I bet the hygienist (and probably the dentist as well) has no idea about the sensitivity and specificity of the test.

Judging from the April 2012 *Choosing Wisely* report from the American Board of Internal Medicine and nineteen specialty boards in conjunction with *Consumer Reports*, ignorance of whether a test or intervention is worthwhile is fairly common.

It found that about 30 percent of tests and interventions done in the U.S. do not benefit the patient (some claim this figure runs as high as 50 percent) and came up with a list of ninety tests that shouldn't be done. It included items like routine annual pap smears on women ages 30 to 65, routine imaging studies on people with low back pain in the first six weeks, routine DEXA scans in women under 65 and men under 70, and electrocardiograms or stress tests in low-risk patients with no symptoms as part of a routine physical (a *Consumer Reports* survey showed 44 percent of respondents had this done).

Many of these interventions were being done inappropriately, and I would hazard a guess they still are. But what concerns me is that so many books giving advice to patients urge them to insist their stupid doctor order lots of tests; what patients really need is an informed doctor ordering the minimum.

Sometimes you don't need tests to diagnose or treat. The minister from the Unitarian Fellowship I associate with had an excoriated, blistery, scaly rash on his arms and was scratching and digging in a very undignified, unministerial way. It looked like poison ivy, but he denied any possible contact.

"It doesn't matter," I told him. "You pretty much treat all itchy rashes the same." He got my "blunderbus" treatment of Prednisone,

Benadryl, and calamine lotion, which treats poison ivy, eczema, insect bites, hives, or whatever it was.

PLAYING DOCTOR YOURSELF

What can you, the emancipated patient, do to ensure your doctor is doing everything necessary to arrive at a correct diagnosis without getting carried away? What can you do to get him to keep an open mind, give adequate considerations to the differential, and order the right tests?

BE A LAB RESULTS READER

It's smart to look at lab results and other records yourself, assuming you have them. If they were sent directly to the doctor's office, request to see them, and get pushy if necessary; don't think that just because it's your body, everyone recognizes your right to unrestricted access. Luckily, though, the Health Insurance Portability and Accountability Act (HIPAA) does, so while you may have to wait and pay a small fee, you can't be refused.

Trisha Torrey's story is a good example of why you should do this. As I said, she was diagnosed with a highly malignant cancer and was on the brink of having some particularly nasty chemo, so she went for a second opinion. She asked that her records be faxed to her to take to the new doctor. When she got them, she started going through them.

She quickly noticed the pathology reports of the biopsy of her lump said "most suspicious for" and "most consistent with" the specific cancer. There was no definitive diagnosis.

Also, because this was a rare cancer (rarity being a sensible trigger for skepticism about a diagnosis), the sample had been sent for further "clonality" testing. These results were not in the chart, and therefore hadn't been seen by the first doctor who was so adamant about the diagnosis and the need for chemo.

When Torrey tracked down the clonality test, lo and behold, it was negative! Her pathology slides were then sent to another pathologist at the National Institute of Health (NIH) who diagnosed her as not having cancer at all, but a benign disease called panniculitis.

Also, sometimes abnormal results get over looked. According to a report in *Archives of Internal Medicine* (November 1999), doctors fail to tell patients about abnormal results one out of fourteen times. The odds may be in your favor, but there's no reason to play them where your health is concerned.

My nephew Michael, a very attentive and emancipated patient with a lot of health concerns, had a CT scan of his chest and an MRI of his head and neck. He emailed me to say he has a "small ductal remnant calcification present" and a "small right maxillary sinus retention cyst." He wanted to know what they meant, since his doctor had completely neglected to mention them.

Fortunately, they didn't mean anything important. On another occasion, he had a sleep study and his doctor didn't tell him anything about the results, and Michael's convinced the doctor didn't even look at them. They showed that in four hours of sleep, he woke up 146 times, often preceded by an unexplained jump in his heart rate. Seems like something worth mentioning.

BE A TEST TESTER

As mentioned, tests are done for various reasons, and not always good ones. Sometimes, your doctor orders too many. Factors like sensitivity and specificity help decide if a test is worthwhile. The hope is that your doctor is sufficiently well informed and ethical to only order tests that are worth doing, but weighing the pros and cons can be complicated, and it's hard for doctors to be sufficiently informed about everything relevant for every test.

Another statistic that helps decide if something is worth doing is called the number needed to treat (NNT). This is an expression of how many patients need to be subject to the intervention for one patient to benefit. It is more often cited for treatments, but the same principle applies to tests.

Mammography seems simple, safe, and benign... a no-brainer even. Why don't we do it on every woman? Because the NNT shows you have to do a mammogram on 2,000 women for ten years for one woman to be saved from breast cancer. What do the other 1,999 women think about having their boobs squished, the radiation exposure, the inconvenience, the expense, and the anxiety, all so that one woman gets diagnosed?

Another stat, sort of opposite of the NNT, is called the number needed to harm (NNH). It offers a tangible measurement of an intervention's downside.

The acclaimed authority on the merits of tests is the U.S. Preventive Services Task Force at www.uspreventiveservices-taskforce.org. It analyzes tests and results and comes up with recommendations, though primarily about the validity of screenings. The Cochrane Collaboration and the Cochrane Library at www.cochrane.org/cochrane-reviews is another useful resource for information about tests.

Frequently, your doctor orders tests because that's just what's done, not knowing the stats. If you ask your doctor to spell out the specificity, sensitivity, NNT, and NNH, you kind of put him on the spot and he may find it difficult to admit he doesn't know. He might then adopt that favorite tactic for avoiding difficult conversations, getting into "busy mode," making the patient feel uncomfortable holding him up by asking all these "silly" questions.

Here are some questions you should get your doctor to answer about tests, which may have more practical value than statistics and are recommended by David H. Newman, M.D., in his book *Hippocrates' Shadow*:

- Is there a clear question the test can answer?
- Is there is a good chance the test will give you a clear yes or no?
- Is there is a plan of action for the result?

The Agency for Healthcare Research and Quality adds:

- What does the test tell?
- What happens if this test is not done now?

- How accurate is it?
- What are the alternatives? Are there safer/cheaper/less uncomfortable ones?
- What happens next?
- Do I need to be prepped for this test in any way?
- When will I get the results?

If your doctor wants a bunch of seemingly unnecessary tests, it can be a bit confrontational to say "No thanks." And there's always the anxiety that you're refusing something that will turn up some vital finding and save your life.

But most doctors won't take umbrage at your questioning the merit of the tests if you approach it in a calm, reasonable way. It's also often a good tactic to suggest a compromise that involves holding off on tests for a little while.

Be A Self-Diagnoser

I'm the first to admit there were cases that had me puzzled that were ultimately solved by the patient. So, if your doctor is having trouble figuring out what's wrong with you, diagnose yourself.

This may prompt you to ask, "Why do I need a doctor at all if he's so lame?" But in all probability, your doctor isn't completely useless and is doing his best, but he needs some help. Rather than usurp his role, you can assist him.

The doctor looks at your symptoms and uses his knowledge of diseases to come up with a differential diagnosis. His knowledge and experience help him draw conclusions about what sort of things are most likely to be wrong with you.

There's a well-worn maxim in medicine to illustrate the profound truth that common things occur commonly. If you ever heard a doctor casually throw in some remark about zebras and wondered what kind of a whacky safari doctor he must be, he was probably referring to this maxim, which goes: "When you hear hoof beats, don't think zebras."

In other words, the most common possibilities are the most likely. Start with them, and save the obscure "zebra" possibilities for when you've ruled out the more likely culprits.

If you're following my advice thus far, you have your test results. This, combined with your intimate knowledge of your symptoms, gives you solid ground on which to base your research.

Various websites provide the relevant information your doctor (hopefully) has in his head already. These can be used to make your own differential diagnosis when you plug in your symptoms. The best of these in my opinion is Isabel System (www.isabelhealthcare.com), followed by i-Triage (www.itriage-health.com). Both provide a list of possible causes for your symptoms and access to information about those conditions.

Incidentally, Isabel System is another good story of medical emancipation and enterprise. Like so many medical self-help books, it was born of a necessity created by a medical crisis and shortcomings of the healthcare system.

When Isabel was 3, she developed chickenpox and took a turn for the worse. It was attributed to the chickenpox at first, but it turned out she had necrotizing fasciitis, a severe infection of the skin and underlying tissues (better known as flesh-eating bacteria) and toxic shock, from which she nearly died.

"Isabel's extensive suffering could have been avoided if the local emergency department and family physicians, instead of assuming her symptoms were typical of the chickenpox from which she was also suffering, had stopped to ask 'what else could this be?'," notes the website.

Her father realized her doctors found it difficult to diagnose something out of the ordinary, as they were always time pressured and some were inexperienced. So he devised an easily searchable database that draws up differential diagnoses from a list of symptoms. It is primarily aimed at doctors, but there's a list patients can access also.

The problem with sites like this—or any other resource, for that matter—is that you're usually confronted with a huge range of possibilities and don't have the knowledge to efficiently weed out the zebras. However, Isabel System does indicates if something is common or not and has a red flag icon on things that are serious.

Trying to diagnose yourself might give you a little empathy for your doctor. This is particularly likely if you have some of those famously vague symptoms like dizziness, weight gain, joint pain, shortness of breath, and abdominal pain, which all have a billion causes.

Fatigue is probably the best of these. As a bit of a lark, I Googled *fatigue*. It got me to E-medicine, which told me, "The majority of illnesses known to man list fatigue." It can be caused by endocrine, kidney, heart, lung, gastrointestinal, psychiatric, or a host of other diseases. It's also an adverse effect of medicines, and often people just aren't getting enough sleep.

Then there are all those conditions that don't cause symptoms, at least not until they're advanced or there's some catastrophic complication. High blood pressure, kidney failure, lots of cancers, and liver failure all may cause no symptoms in early stages; often, coronary artery disease presents for the first time with a possibly lethal heart attack.

The bottom line is, it may be worth investigating your illness if your doctor has difficulty arriving at a diagnosis that makes sense or that appropriate treatments aren't managing. Just be sure to use only reputable sources, which is something I talk about more in *Getting the Right Information*. In case you haven't heard, there's a lot of garbage on the internet.

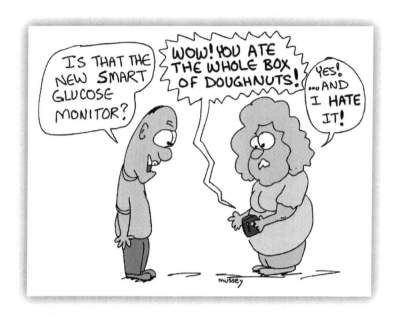

Be A DIYer

In this day and age, you can order lab tests for yourself at My Lab Test (www.mylabtest.com). You just have to know what to order, the appropriate ICD code, and how to interpret the results. But this can be a useful option for some follow-up tests, like rechecking thyroid levels, your Hemoglobin A1c if you are diabetic, or your cholesterol, when the results should be straightforward.

Be Skeptical

Sometimes patients have hard-to-diagnose conditions and the doctor never pins down an exact diagnosis. He has to fly by the seat of his pants, saying lame things like, "It doesn't have the feel of something sinister." But this is unsatisfactory, and it's not unreasonable to be skeptical.

Questioning your doctor is perfectly legitimate. But I know from experience that assertive patients can come across a little threatening and distrustful, so be kind, gracious, and reasonable.

The self-help advocates strongly encourage skepticism, especially if the diagnosis is unusual. Be skeptical if you've never heard of what your doctor is diagnosing, if you're not getting better, if the diagnosis doesn't ring true or jibe with what you read ("Trust your instincts," Torrey says), and especially if it's based on just one test.

Often, that one test is some radiological study the doctor hangs his diagnostic hat on. "Currently, the average diagnostic error in interpreting medical images is in the 20 percent to 35 percent range," warns Eshan Samei from the Advanced Imaging Laboratory at Duke University Medical Center.

Current techniques, like CTs and MRIs, generate hundreds or thousands of images for the radiologist to review. It's not like the old days, when a chest X-ray consisted of one film looking from back to front and one looking from the side. Now, if an ER doctor orders a CT scan to chekc for appendicitis, for example, the radiologist has hundreds of images to look at, and very probably has films from all sorts of other acute cases and train wrecks vying for his attention. It's easy to miss stuff or get something wrong.

Smart skeptical questions for your doctor include:

- What else could it be? What's the worst thing it could be?
- How confident are you in the diagnosis?

- Are there findings/symptoms that don't fit your diagnosis?
- What further tests might be helpful?
- What's my prognosis?
- What organizations and resources do you recommend for support and information?

This may shake a complacent doctor out of his reverie, or out of bad cognitive habits like anchoring.

The arch cynics would point out that with a fee-for-service payment system, there's no incentive for doctors to make diagnosis and get patients better. But hopefully yours isn't so wantonly profiteering. Most doctors try their best to help patients in the face of many obstacles. And most should appreciate your informed involvement in the difficult business of making a diagnosis.

WHEN YOUR DOCTOR THINKS YOU'RE CRAZY

Functional/psychosomatic/psychological/somatoform disorder diagnoses warrant special attention. These refer to a psychological component to whatever ails you, which is incredibly common. Often, this sort of diagnosis leads to misunderstanding, with the patient believing the doctor is dismissing him as crazy. This can be the kiss of death for further cooperation between doctor and patient.

As a great example of this kind of misunderstanding, listen to Torrey, who's usually so reasonable:

"Are there patients who imagine their symptoms and only crave the attention their symptoms might bring? I suppose there are. But my educated guess says that the doctor, unable to assign a name to the ailment, is looking to place the blame on the patient, and not on his own inability to do his job."

One fallacy is the idea that the patient is imagining symptoms and acting intentionally, capriciously, to gain attention. Another is that the doctor invokes a psychological element from the inability to find out what's "really" wrong.

Psychological stuff can produce real symptoms and real illnesses. The human brain is a powerful organ.

I used a variety of terms for the psychological element because there are many, which is part of the problem, but the most precise is "somatoform disorder." This refers to a tendency of psychological stresses to manifest as physical symptoms (or to use the more lyrical description of pioneering British psychiatrist Sir Henry Maudsley, "The sorrow that has no vent in tears may make other organs weep").

The name has changed again, though, with the newest edition of the Diagnostic and Statistical Manual. Now it's "somatic symptom disorder," presumably so it can have a snappy acronym like SSD.

Whatever you call it, it is very real and not a deliberate contrivance of the patient. It's also a fallacy to assume once a doctor has decided someone has some psychopathology, he ignores other issues, gives up looking for anything else, blows the patient off, and moves on to some respectably sane patient.

That would probably close his practice, since in my experience, all patients are a little screwy. But then, so are all the doctors.

It's nonsense to think of the brain as separate from the body. Yet that's been the tradition, separating mental and physical illnesses, and people often see it as an either/or situation.

Somatoform disorders often manifest with neurological symptoms (e.g., numbness, tingling, dizziness, headaches), gastrointestinal symptoms (like cramping, bloating, variations in bowel movements), and sexual dysfunction. Or, the bugbear of so many doctors, chronic pain, because it's often associated with narcotic use and possible abuse.

The main hurdle is there's no blood test or imaging technique to confirm a somatoform disorder diagnosis. It's a diagnosis of exclusion, meaning it's the doctor's job to diligently rule out physical or organic causes.

Even now, I'm talking about this in an either/or context. Somatoform or physical. But in nearly all patients, there's a bit of both. Maybe it's arthritis of the neck with muscle spasms made worse by stress. Maybe it's irritable bowel syndrome aggravated by anxiety or depression; any kind of pain tends to get worse with depression. Maybe it's high blood pressure or heart arrhythmias made worse by mania.

Ulcers, hypertension, headaches, asthma... there's a long list of problems associated with or exacerbated by stress and anxiety. This is the same as talking about somatoform disorders and psychological factors. Somehow, though, it seems more acceptable to many folks to say an illness was "aggravated by stress" than to imply depression or a psychosomatic component was responsible.

Anyone who's sick is likely to be anxious about it, especially if the doctor can't find a cause.

Hypochondriasis is a variation on this. It's an anxiety disorder involving an obsession with any kind of illness or symptom. The anxiety goes beyond what's justified. Headaches are indicative of a brain tumor; numbness and tingling mean multiple sclerosis; bouts of diarrhea are from colon cancer; chest pain is a heart attack; and so on. It's incredibly difficult to get such patients to accept that their problems may be mainly somatoform, not physical.

Distinguishing between somatoform and organic illnesses or symptoms can be a challenge. When tests keep coming up normal; when symptoms never progress to some clear diagnosis; when there are indications of stress or psychiatric conditions like depression, anxiety, thought disorder, sleep disturbance, or substance abuse; these factors tend to point to a psychological element, which may be the sole problem or aggravating a "real" problem.

A Tale With A Point

Here I am upbraiding the medical profession for doing too many tests, but the story of Canadian Billy McNeely, reported by the BBC, suggests that sometimes doctors don't do enough.

McNeely was involved in a brawl in 2010 after an arm wrestling bout, and he was stabbed five times. He was sewn up at the local hospital, but continued to suffer itching and pain in his back, which was attributed to nerve damage. He also noted, "I've done some jail time in the past," and "the guards rub you over with a metal wand detector, and every time it hit my back … it went off."

Three years later, when he was scratching his back, his fingernail caught on something. He had his girlfriend look and she told him, "There's a knife blade sticking out of your back."

A 3-inch knife blade was removed. This prompted Billy to chastise—and threaten to sue—the doctors, saying "They should've X-rayed right off in the beginning."

GETTING A SECOND OPINION

When your doctor can't make a diagnosis, or you suspect it's wrong, or you aren't getting better, get a second opinion. Your doctor might see this as a no-confidence vote, but hopefully he'll happily share the wealth and be relieved to have some help; he might even suggest it himself.

In *YOU: The Smart Patient*, the authors say to always get a second opinion, noting, "Research has found that getting a second opinion results in a new diagnosis in as many as 30 percent of all cases."

Always getting a second opinion seems a little over the top, especially if you're dealing with some minor illness. But deciding what's serious enough to warrant it is sometimes a difficult call. It largely depends on how much faith you have in your doctor.

A second opinion is important when surgery, chemotherapy, or some other risky or radical treatment is proposed. Also, if your diagnosis is something obscure, have someone else weigh in.

In *Doctor, Your Patient Will See You Now*, Kussin advises skepticism whenever you're seeing a doctor with some vested interest—usually financial—in the treatment he recommends for your diagnosis.

For example, get a second opinion when an orthopedic surgeon presses for a joint replacement and he has a financial relationship with the manufacturer of the prosthesis. Get a second opinion when a doctor suggests treatment with a particular medicine and he has a financial relationship with the drug company (Kussin cites a study in the *New England Journal of Medicine*, noting 94 percent of physicians have relationships with pharmaceutical and medical device companies).

If your doctor sends you to a surgeon for an operation or an oncologist for chemo, make the most of the extra appointment. Don't just use a specialist as a mechanic; bring all your records and have him review your diagnosis. Ask for his specialized knowledge to confirm your doctor got it right. This doesn't only provide a second opinion, it forces the specialist to stop and think instead of treating on autopilot.

CHAPTER 3

GETTING THE RIGHT INFORMATION

———— ◆ ————

THE TRUTH IS OUT THERE

MY WIFE PAULA AND I kept running into this hippie-looking couple at every party, reception, and social event we attended around town. We started referring to them as "our new best friends," even though we didn't know their names.

Eventually, we learned their names, and like a self-fulfilling prophecy, Lynne and Ernie are now best friends of ours.

One day, Ernie e-mailed me to say they found a lump on his kidney. He asked what it might be, what the best treatment would be, and who the best person to see would be. The main concern, obviously, was whether it was cancer.

Not unreasonable questions, and the sort you expect your doctor to be able to answer. As a primary care doctor, you'd think I could answer them and advise any patient with such questions. But I didn't know everything there is to know about kidney lumps.

As an exercise I thought useful for this book, I decided to play patient, rather than resorting to what a primary care doctor would normally do in this situation: refer to a specialist. I went to Google and entered *kidney lump* and got a pretty comprehensive list of causes from www.rightdiagnosis.com. Mostly, I wanted to explore the possibility of cancer, though.

The site gives the basic rundown on kidney cancer. It also lists conditions that can mimic the symptoms, a nice touch.

Narrowing the search, I went to www.kidneycancer.org for more in-depth stuff on types of cancers, how they're diagnosed, and the treatments. The site told me renal cell carcinoma is by far the most common type of cancer affecting the kidneys. It also clearly explains the staging process that assesses how far the cancer has advanced.

I also looked at the Mayo Clinic site, which gives more detailed information about RCC, to use the abbreviation that lets everyone know you're no novice. This site also has a physician finder tool for a specialist in kidney cancer, though there were none listed close to me.

So I tried to find a specialist using the trick described in *Getting the Right Doctor*, looking at the authors of recent research papers on Google Scholar for a name that crops up repeatedly. In this instance, Robert Motzer from Memorial Sloan-Kettering Cancer Center in New York City was one.

Everyone's case is different, of course, and Ernie was likely going to need a specialist or two (probably first a urologist, then an oncologist if the mass looked like cancer), a biopsy, and possibly a staging workup. But just knowing RCC was a primary concern, what the appropriate diagnostic course of action was, and what the treatment options might be put Ernie in a good position to oversee what happened next.

The level of sophistication you can acheive doing your own research is impressive, judging by a story I came accross from two Australian researchers looking at the idea of doctors using the internet to make diagnoses. In the Novemebr 2006 *British Medical Journal*, they say, "It seems that patients use Google to diagnose their own medical disorders too" (probably a more novel idea back in 2006).

They tell of a 16-year-old water polo player who presented with acute subclavian vein thrombosis, or clotting in one of the large veins in the arm pit.

One researcher was explaining to the patient and his dad that it was hard to know why a thrombosis had developed. The patient's father jumped in, saying, "He has Paget-Schrötter syndrome," a very rare condition where repetitive arm motions lead to thrombosis in the vein.

The father had simply Googled the symptoms, he explained to the dumbfounded researchers. He then gave them "a mini-tutorial on the pathophysiology ... and told us the correct treatment."

Information is empowering. But the big problem is knowing where to get it.

THE EMPOWERING INFORMATION AGE

In the good old days, the doctor was perceived to know all about what was wrong with you, and it was an image he worked hard to project and protect.

Lay folk couldn't access or understand the sources of information—medical textbooks and journals—and it was kind of like the Middle Ages, when the priest was the only person considered capable of interpreting the Bible. You came before the doctor, bowing and tugging your forelock, hanging on his every word, not knowing enough to question his proclamations.

But now the information age has leveled the playing field. Today, patients can know as much as their doctors, at least about their own specific issues. This puts them in a better position to be in charge of their health and make decisions about care that reflect their own values and opinions.

There are so many medical websites, second only to the number of porn sites. As of early 2014, WebMD was averaging 156 million unique visitors per month and almost 13 billion annual page views.

"Up to 80 percent of internet users report they have sought medical information online," says *Scientific American* website Pathways in a September 2010 article. It also notes two-thirds of patients want their doctors to recommend reliable online resources.

Emphasising the need to be selective, Dr. Paula Cundy, chairman of the British Medical Association's technology subcommittee, notes that while there's much more information available than ever before, a lot of it "is seriously wrong."

TMI

"TMI" and "eeeuuuuwww, Dad" are typically what you hear from your kids if you start talking about having sex with their mother or some other sensitive or "inappropriate" subject. But in the medical world, too much information is a literal problem. It's impossible to know all about everything, to keep up with the latest developments in every field, to know the best tests and treatments and specialists, etc.

More so than the information age, we are in the TMI age. From the dawn of mankind to 2003, we accumulated a measly one billion GB (that's ten-to-the-9th gigabytes) of information. But now, we're talking zettabytes (ten-to-the-12th, or one trillion GB) and we're accumulating several zettabytes of information each year.

This is paralleled in the medical world. A 2010 article in *PLOS Medicine* notes there are now seventy-five trials and eleven systemic reviews of trials published *each day*. There are some 500 medical journals churning out about one million articles per year.

No doctor can keep up, which is why I've always had to explain to my patients, using one of my favorite turgid maxims, that "I'm a Jack-of-all-trades, and master of none." I tell them that's why god invented specialists, the experts who focus on particular chunks of anatomy or conditions.

Even they are becoming more narrowly focused these days. And even they struggle to keep up and have their limitations.

My friend Ernie also had a prostate cancer and was all lined up to have a radical prostatectomy. But with his own online research, he learned of a specialized treatment technique used in some centers. An MRI scan of the prostate is performed using a radionuclide enhancement, which his urologist hadn't offered as an option and appeared to not even know about.

The MRI showed the cancer to be localized to one small area of the prostate. He and his urologist decided it was not necessary to operate at this point and instead continue "watchful waiting."

Your ultimate safeguard is to be sufficiently well informed to oversee your healthcare and guide your doctor. It's sort of a theme of this book, if you haven't noticed.

KNOW-IT-ALL DOCS DON'T KNOW IT ALL

To stress the point, it's naïve and potentially dangerous to simply assume your doctor has all the best, most accurate, most up-to-date information.

"The dirty little secret about medicine is that we physicians make decisions all the time based on woefully incomplete information," claims Stanford cardiologist Paula Yock, writing in the April 2009 edition of *The Economist*.

Ideally, doctors should pay attention to best practices, those guidelines put together by experts in consideration of all the studies on a given subject. But this is pie in the sky to a large extent. As noted in *Getting the Right Diagnosis*, so much is done by rote or by that's-how-it's-always-been-done thinking, and often this is without factual backup.

Your doctor needs a sufficient fund of knowledge to differentiate a cold from strep throat or a migraine from a tension headache and to know who should get a PSA test (no one?), which depressed patients are at increased risk of suicide, whether to order a CT scan or an X-ray for your sinus pain, which imaging studies to order for lower back pain, and what medicines to prescribe for your first bout of Herpes. There's an endless list of things you need to know to be a competent doctor.

But not every doctor is a gem. Plus, as you'll see in depth in *Getting the Right Treatment*, doctors get fed a lot of biased information by drug companies.

It's a delicate issue to find out if your doctor is well informed. It will not endear you if you march in and ask "Do you know what you're doing?"

Use the advice in *Getting the Right Doctor* to check out the competence of a potential provider. Look for doctors using electronic health records, as they are most likely to have easiest access to information and should be using the newest objective guidelines.

Check out best practices for yourself to see if your doctor is doing the right things. Go to the DHSS's National Guideline Clearing House (www.guidelines.gov), the American College of Physicians (www.acponline.org), or The Cochrane Reviews.

INTIMIDATING OR OVERWHELMING YOUR DOCTOR

An empowered patient loaded with information can be threatening to a doctor and brusing to his ego. It's scary when patients think of themselves as equals and question decisions. And certainly many doctors have a bad habit of making unilateral decisions.

But keep in mind that even with your profound knowledge, you have something of a myopic view of a very narrow slice of medical wisdom. That doesn't mean you necessarily have a good grasp of the big picture, which is an important part of care.

In Ernie's case, for example, if he had coronary artery disease or a coagulopathy, it must be considered when deciding whether to operate or not. Although Ernie might have become a leading expert on prostate cancer, he might not be all that well informed about the dangers of having a heart attack or bleeding to death during surgery.

A variation on TMI is when patients come in with too much information. The typical nightmare scenario is a hypochondriacal patients shouldering his or her way into the consulting room with a huge sheaf of printouts under the arm, expecting the doctor to wade through it all.

If the information is misleading or just downright wrong, it takes twice as long to disabuse someone of mistaken notions than it does to give them the strait dope in the first place. That's not conducive to a beneficial appointment, given its invariably very limited time.

Dr. Scott Haig published an article called "When Your Patient Is a Googler" in a 2007 *TIME*. It's fairly indicative of the hostility emancipated, empowered, self-sufficient patients can generate in the medical profession. He describes such patients as "suspicious and distrustful, their pressured sentences bursting with misused, mispronounced words and half-baked ideas." Much of the article was, of course, dismissed by the laypeople in the online comments as "a scathingly arrogant attack" and the like.

Don't be deterred. There's too much on the line.

WHERE TO GO TO KNOW

It's impossible to be a proactive, emancipated participant in your healthcare without sources of reliable information about your medical conditions.

One thing that makes gathering good information so difficult—for doctors as well as patients—is that things change all the time, and rapidly. Medicine is famous for U-turns. The hottest intervention or advice today is all wrong tomorrow.

There's the old-fashioned stuff like bloodletting, murcury, and phosphorus, all of which turned out to be positivly murderous. Now, low-fat diets are not the pinnacle of healthy eating; today it's low-carb diets. Saturated fat was absolute taboo a few years ago, now it's OK. The FDA has just reversed itself on recomendations to limit seafood in kids and pregnant women, now believing the omega-3 benefits outweigh the mercury risk. Even without complete reversals, many modifications take place all the time. Along with it all, websites come and go with amazing speed.

The takeaway is the need for current information. Not that there's any guarantee it'll be good next month, but it's the best you can hope for. When evaluating information, check its date. Information tends to sit around for a long time, especially online. And this prompts a disclaimer that the websites I talk about below may change between my writing and your reading.

The Internet

Most internet users look for health information online, and 75 percent of them use what they find to make medical decisions, according to Steven Kussin, M.D. He also says only four of the top 100 medical websites meet all four criteria for accuracy outlined by the *Journal of the American Medical Association* (*JAMA*).

JAMA has further complicated things. It found that just because the attributed author of online content has medical credentials, it doesn't mean the content is accurate.

So, the big question is: How do you find reliable sites?

A significant factor in assessing objectivity is to know if the site has a particular vested interest or sponsorship. There are diabetic sites run by drug companies that sell insulin, for example. LillyDiabetes (www.lillydiabetes.com) is one.

It's likely such a site will not be enthusiastic about non-pharmacological treatments like diet and exercise. Such a site probably wouldn't subscribe to the idea that resorting to insulin is a bit of a failure of lifestyle changes. "Starting insulin is a smart step toward good health," says the Lilly site, "not a sign of failure."

Other respectable sites, though not owned by any particular merchant, may still be a bit promotional. One of the most popular medical sites, WebMD, has ads for Claritin on its allergy page, for example. It seems to me, as happens even in the most respectable medical journals, the sponsorship of advertisers could influence the editorial content of the site.

"The predatory dynamic should always be kept in mind," warns Eric Topol, M.D.

The National Center for Complementary and Integrative Health (NCCIH) at nccih.nih.gov (which was, until recently adopting newly favored terminology, the National Center for Complementary and Alternative Medicine) offers good advice for assessing health information websites. "It costs money to run a website," it explains, but who sponsors the site is important in assessing objectivity. "You should know how the site pays for its existence. Does it sell advertising? Is it sponsored by a drug company?"

NCCIH also recommends favoring URLs that end in .gov, indicating a government-sponsored site, or .edu, denoting an educational institiution. While .org used to reliably indicate a noncommercial site, that's no longer the case.

The Health on the Net Foundation (www.hon.ch), a Swiss-based organization "founded to encourage the dissemination of quality health information for patients and professionals and the general public," can help you find quality medical websites. HON provides certification to sites that meet its criteria, so look for the HONcode logo. Click on it and you should be taken to the HON home site to confirm the status of the website you're interested in.

Kussin says the "hands down, thumbs up best free public domain site" is UpToDate at www.uptodate.com. It provides free basic information for patients or more specialized information for paid subscribers. Healthcare professionals might want a full subscription, but you can join temporarily while you research your particular subject. At the time of this writing, it's $19.95 for seven days or $44.95 for 30 days.

Net Top 20 (medical.nettop20.com) ranks medical websites, which might also help. Incidentally, the top two sites on their list are WebMD (www.webmd.com) and HealthCentral (www.healthcentral.com).

Worth a specific mention is the site iTriage (www.itriage-health.com), as it's a good tool for making a diagnosis with its easy-to-use and comprehensive symptom checker, complete with cell phone app. It also helps you find providers and learn about healthcare and procedures.

For more serious academic sites that provide highly technical information, two respected resources are:

The National Center for Biotechnology Information's site, PubMed (www.pubmed.gov), the largest component of which is Medline (www.medlineplus.gov). It's a "freely accessible online database of biomedical journal citations and abstracts created by the U.S. National Library of Medicine." They index "approximately 5,400 journals published in the United States and more than 80 other countries." See why doctors have such a hard time keeping up?

The Cochrane Collaboration and the Cochrane Library (www.cochrane.org/cochrane-reviews), a network of more than 28,000 people from over 100 countries reviewing all the high-quality evidence on a particular healthcare subject and then publishing their conclusions. It's a good resource for guidance on what are and are not valid treatments, tests, and interventions.

To date, Cochrane has published over 5,000 reviews to help guide doctors, policymakers, and patients. "Our work is internationally recognised as the benchmark for high quality information about the effectiveness of health care," the site modestly proclaims. Cochrane does seem to be universally acknowledged as the definitive opinion, though.

The Cochrane Library also curates Central, the largest collection of randomized controlled trials in the world.

Both PubMed and the Cochrane Collaboration are high-quality academic sites. The problem is they are both so large and comprehensive that it's a challenge navigating them.

The information, though of high quality, tends to be technical and may be hard to understand. The boffins that write this stuff have a special stylized language that almost seems intended to obfuscate.

It can be difficult to get answers to specific questions. You often have to read around the subject and make your best judgment. If you're wondering whether your thyroid could be abnormal even though a blood test says it's not, you have to read about thyroid and the blood test and put it all together.

Google Scholar gives you access to a lot of original papers and learned articles.

As with so many sites these days, you may have to sign up, which can be a pain, and always presents a concern about what the site will do with your information. And sometimes you have to pay, as is often the case to get a full article on PubMed.

For information about medicines, the online version of the *Physicians' Desk Reference* at www.pdr.net and Epocrates at www.epocrates.com are good resources.

If you're looking to buy medicines online (covered in more depth in *Getting the Right Price*), my top choice for guidance is the Consumer Reports information on Where to Buy Your Medicines. For information about alternative medicines and treatments, go to the NCCIH site.

Specialized societies and organizations focused on a particular illness are often good resources, too. For example, there's the

American Cancer Society at www.cancer.org or more narrow-ly focused groups like the National Breast Cancer Foundation at www.nationalbreastcancer.org. There's the Alzheimers Foundation of America at www.alzfdn.org and the National Multiple Sclerosis Society at www.nationalmssociety.org, and so on. Sites like those run by the American Heart Association at www.heart.org and the National Institute of Diabetes and Digestive and Kidney Diseases at www.niddk.nih.gov are other solid sources of information.

If you're trying to get the latest dope on research in a par-ticular medical field, www.clinicaltrials.gov tells you about on-going or recently completed clinical trials.

The Patient Advocate Foundation (www.patientadvocate.org) is a go-to resource for information about health insurance. It also has a lot of other information to help with many aspects of your healthcare.

SOCIAL MEDIA SITES
Social media websites like Facebook, Twitter, and Google+ ob-viously aren't medical sites, but they can be a good resource. Deborah Kogan says Facebook saved her son's life.

Four-year-old Leo Kogan got sick with a rash, fever, and fa-cial swelling. He was diagnosed with scarlet fever (an illness as-sociated with strep throat) and put on amoxicillin. His progress was slow and his mother posted a picture of him with his very swollen face on Facebook, talking about how sick he still was and his persistent fever.

Within minutes she got a call from an ex-neighbor. She said her son Max had the exact same thing and was diagnosed and hospitalized with Kawasaki's disease, a nasty autoimmune condition that attacks the liver and coronary arteries. Deborah took Leo to the hospital, and sure enough, he had Kawasaki's and some liver damage already.

Writing on Slate.com, she gives credit to the benefit of social media, with the title "How Facebook Saved My Son's Life."

In the wake of Web 2.0, driven more by user-generated content and social media than by static web pages, comes the so-called Health 2.0 evolution.

Blogs, forums, message boards, wikis, video sites, and other mediums allow people to share and compare experiences. Patients Like Me (www.patientslikeme.com) is a popular site founded by Jamie Heywood, whose brother had Amyotrophic Lateral Sclerosis (ALS, otherwise known as Lou Gehrig's disease). "We have learned so much about what patients need to know. We hope to help patients share their knowledge with others," says Heywood.

Much of what is shared is subjective thoughts and feelings. Without wishing to sound negative, you have to maintain a degree of skepticism and judge the quality of any information being shared. But there are also great opportunitites for users to learn from each other, and even to interact with trained professionals.

Books

Apart from the internet, there are a few printed resources worthy of mention, though they all have online editions. Despite being large, cumbersome, impractical, dreary tomes, these reference books have their places in the history and folklore of medical practice and are still used by some (usually as little as possible).

The *Physicians' Desk Reference* (PDR) is an unwieldy compendium of 3,480 pages of package inserts. It's probably the best known of these dinosaurs.

Package inserts are what the manufacturers issue with each of their products. This is an almost incomprehensible list of properties of the drug, manufacturing details, adverse effects, dosing schedules, etc. They are crammed with so much irrelevant information, it's almost impossible to figure out something basic like the standard dosage.

If you're in danger of getting a hernia from taking out the PDR, go to www.pdr.net. There's also a *PDR Family Guide for Prescription Drugs*.

Then there's the *International Statistical Classification of Disease* (ICD). I know, it should be *ISCD*, but somehow the *S* got lost. And there's the *Current Procedural Terminology* code book (*CPT*). Both are about as exciting as the *PDR*, containing a list of everything you can have wrong with you, with a number allocated to each. Both are upgraded periodically and the current versions are online.

The *Diagnostic and Statistical Manual of Mental Disorders* (*DSM*) is much more often used by the lay public. I consider it a reflection of our society's fascination with and poor understanding of mental illness. Check it out online at dsm.psychiatryonline.org or shell out $199 for your own hardcopy at www.appi.org/Home.

Cartoonist Ellen Forney was diagnosed as bipolar shortly before her thirtieth birthday. Flagrantly manic, she likened herself to other artists and writers who suffered from mood disorders, like Vincent van Gogh, Georgia O'Keeffe, William Styron, and Sylvia Plath. She was terrified that medications would cause her to lose creativity, questioning whether an artist's bipolar disorder is a curse or a gift.

At first, she didn't believe her psychiatrist's diagnosis. He showed her the *DSM* and "We went through the symptoms together," she related in an NPR interview. "It was just a very, very strange, strange feeling to see what I had thought of—in particular when I was manic—as super-duper me; exponentially me; very, very, very me, and to see it right there in a book."

She wrote a rather wacky cartoon narrative about her experience, *Marbles: Mania, Depression, Michelangelo, and Me.*

The fourth book worth a mention is the *Merck Manual of Diagnosis and Therapy*, better known as just the *Merck Manual*, "the worlds best-selling medical textbook," according to

Wikipedia. It was first published in 1899 and is now in its eleventh edition. There's also a *Home Health Handbook* for patients and caregivers, and even the *Merck Manual for Pet Health*.

These are available online at the Merck website, www.merckmanuals.com, and there's even an app version for your cell phone.

JOURNALS AND TEXTBOOKS

Medical journals and textbooks are other hardcopy references, once the principal resources for people looking up medical information.

Augusto and Michaela Odone, the parents of Lorenzo Odone (of Lorenzo's Oil fame), proved the usefulness of these resources. They came up with a life saving—or life prolonging—treatment for Lorenzo after hours of digging through research papers in journals.

Lorenzo had a horrible neuro-degenerative disease (adrenoleukodystrophy, or ALD). All the doctors said he was going to die and there was nothing they could do about it. In desperation, they scoured textbooks and journals at the nearby NIH library in Chevy Chase, trying to find some cure.

They wore themselves to a frazzle, but finally came across an obscure research paper from a Polish team who noted they were able to lower the level of the toxic long-chain fatty acids that were poisoning Lorenzo's nerves with extra unsaturated fatty acids. They are the basis of the dietary supplement they fed him, which became known as Lorenzo's Oil.

It's another of those great stories of patient self-sufficiency.

There are many medical textbooks. Some are generalized (*Harrison's Principals of Internal Medicine* was always my favorite) and others cover specialized subjects like endocrinology, neurology, orthopedics, general surgery, psychiatry, etc.

And there are billions of journals. These too come generalized, as with the most popular ones like *JAMA*, *The British Medical Journal*, and *The New England Journal of Medicine* (*NEJM*). Then there are one or more journals for every specialty you can think of, and many that you can't.

A large public library may carry some of these. Otherwise, local hospitals often have medical libraries with at least some of the more popular journals. Medical schools are a good resource, too. Nowadays, many of the papers appearing in journals are available on the particular journal's website, but you may have to pay for the privilege of seeing them in their entirety.

However, as I'll get into in *Getting the Right Treatment*, there is a good deal of skepticism about the objectivity of some of the clinical trials and information published in medical journals these days. There are plenty of accusations and some evidence that the editorial content is sometimes unduly influenced by advertisers.

In general, journals are a good resource if you want cutting-edge information about a specialized subject, while textbooks offer a slightly broader picture. You may encounter some difficulty deciphering all the jargon, though; websites are often more friendly to lay readers.

Again I'll stress the importance of checking publication dates. Things move fast and printed resources aren't quite as easily and efficiently updated as those online.

DIG THE DIGITAL

Now to shift gears away from research and general information. The information you and your doctor have about your medical history is an entirely different aspect of this chapter. And again, computers and technology play crucial roles in accessing, disseminating, and processing information.

The field of health information technology (HIT) is defined by the U.S. Department of Health and Human Services as "The application of information processing involving both computer hardware and software that deals with the storage, retrieval, sharing, and use of healthcare information, data, and knowledge for communication and decision making."

Basically, HIT is the overarching system of digitized medicine. On a smaller scale, individual doctors and practices are increasingly using computerized electronic health or medical records (EHRs/EMRs). These refer to a computerized system of storing and sharing charts and other information instead of relying on some massive, disintegrating, overstuffed, illegible paper folders, as has traditionally been the case with medical records.

There's been a lot of reluctance and foot dragging about implementing EHRs. InformationWeek's site Healthcare (www.informationweek.com/healthcare.asp) said in July 2010 that less than 20 percent of the 700,000 practicing doctors were using EHR. Promisingly, though, the CDC reports that by July 2012, 55 percent of doctors and practices were on board.

Still, following a review of the Medicare and Medicaid Services data on meaningful use, it was reported in the February 2013 *NEJM* that only one in six doctors has adopted EHR to the extent of being eligible for a meaningful-use bonus.

While it all seems great (in theory at least), as things gradually go digital, there are not-unreasonable concerns about privacy. Some people worry about having their most intimate medical secrets flung into cyberspace. But all the involved vendors swear their systems are super secure and hacker-proof.

COMPUTERS TO THE RESCUE(?)

Computers accomplish many things.

They will do away with paper charts. Long-term and medically complicated patients tend to accumulate large, unwieldy charts in which it's impossible to find anything. I have an enduring image of my friend and colleague Russell, an arch procrastinator who'd always be behind on his lab reviews and messages, sitting at a desk piled so high with charts he couldn't be seen behind them.

To share any information, these ungainly things have to be disseminated by the outdated business of photocopying and mailing or faxing. And, despite their bulk, they have an impressive knack for getting lost around the office.

Computerized records are not only more manageable, they also have the merit of being legible, unlike any doctor's handwritten Sanskrit notes. It's a serious issue; a July 2006 report by the Institute of Medicine claims doctor handwriting kills more than 7,000 people annually. Illegible prescriptions are largely to blame, and e-scripts will obviate all that. The pharmacist soon won't be wondering whether it says Voltaren or Vytorin, Adderal or Inderal.

EHRs can include built-in alerts so doctors don't make dumb mistakes like prescribing something someone is allergic to or medicines that interact with each other. Such things are all too easy to overlook.

Computers are also good at keeping track of things like when you're due for your next hemoglobin A1c test, pneumonia shot, pap smear, colonoscopy, mammogram, or whatever. This is where computerization is likely to lead to an overall improvement of preventive care and, in the long run, savings on the runaway cost of healthcare.

The connectivity of computers is a key part of their benefits. Once online, doctors can instantly send information to pharmacists, other doctors for referrals, testing facilities, insurance companies, regulatory agencies, or interested parties like the health department to tell them about a notifiable disease like syphilis. The sky's the limit. This greatly increases practice efficiency and reduces payroll costs. Doctors can even easily send helpful stuff like educational materials and detailed prescription information to patients.

The only proviso is the required "interoperability." That's a bit of an issue, but more on it soon.

Computerization also allows for email communication to make appointments, request information, or, if the doctor's practice is really in the space age, for the patient to communicate directly with the doctor. Often, an actual office visit doesn't seem necessary, with an e-mail sufficing to let the doctor know what your blood pressure is, for example.

One study by Kaiser found a 26 percent reduction in office visits with use of email, though others have shown an increase in office visits in practices who had email access. If the latter is true, it may be because important things come to the doctor's attention more readily, which is a good thing.

A major deterrent to email consults is that insurance companies, in their wisdom, won't pay for them. And doctors have this unreasonable desire to get paid for their services.

This might be changing, though. BlueCross BlueShield, through their subsidiary WellPoint, has several pilot programs using RelayHealth (a company promoting innovative health information technologies), and BlueShield of California started an email consult program for its members. So, it may be that common sense will prevail in the end, and insurance companies will adopt a policy of paying for email consults.

When everyone else in the world is using email to communicate efficiently, you might wonder what's wrong with the medical profession.

What's wrong is that medicine is still predominantly in the pre-internet era.

Having a nationwide (or even worldwide) HIT system is anticipated to have multiple benefits. It's expected to reduce healthcare costs by increasing administrative efficiency, help disseminate and promote best practices, better monitor chronic disease, expand access to affordable care, and significantly improve big-picture surveillance of evolving disease trends (like flu outbreaks or a high prevalence of cancers from some local carcinogen). A HIT system should also more efficiently pick up on adverse drug effects; it may have more quickly caught on to the increase in heart attacks caused by the arthritis drug Vioxx, for example.

The proof is in the pudding, as they say. The VA was one of the first to adopt an EHR system, and its medication error rate is seven per one million prescriptions. In the U.S. overall, the rate is 7,000 times higher! At the Brigham and Woman's Hospital, EHR precipitated a 41 percent reduction in error rate and a 51 percent reduction in adverse drug reactions, notes Topol.

TEACHING OLD DOCS NEW TRICKS

Of course, there's the problem of teaching a bunch of conservative old-dog doctors new tricks. It is tough and requires a lot of adaptation in a population who finds digital medicine about as appealing as a prostate exam.

It's disruptive. I've felt the effects when picking up extra shifts at the clinic when some spazzed out, overwhelmed colleague decides he just can't deal with coming in and volunteering for the evening after a day of fighting with the computer.

When writing a piece about the hardships of implementation for my newspaper, I wanted to speak to local friend and colleague Mat Hengy, who was in the process of converting. I called the office. "We've been live for two weeks," his harried-sounding wife/office manager Kena told me.

It was 9.30 p.m. before Mat finished the nightly chore of data entry and was finally able to call me back and give me an earful of his personal reflections on the matter.

Like so many others wedded to the old days, he claims, "I had a great system with paper charts ... with easy-to-find medicine lists and problem lists and stuff highlighted in yellow that needed to be followed up on. Now I have to go through multiple screens to get the information I want."

Changing over is expensive. *InformationWeek* reports a cost of $30,000 per community doctor and $100,000 per bed for hospitals. The American Recovery and Reinvestment Act does provide assistance of $44,000 per eligible doctor through Medicare and $63,750 through Medicaid paid over ten years.

There are strings attached, however. To be eligible, your EHR system has to be capable of "meaningful use." That includes things like maintaining medication and problem lists, checking for potential drug adverse effects, providing patients with a clinical summary of office visits, recording demographics, and being capable of information exchange among providers.

Along with this carrot, there's also a stick. EHR is mandatory as of 2014, and there are financial penalties after 2015 for noncompliance.

Doctors aren't famous for being on the cutting edge of technology. Many don't type, at least not with more than two index fingers. EHR companies have tried to accommodate with special pens they claim can read even doctors' handwritten notes and with the always-imperfect voice recognition software. The website LiveJournal reports on the problem of "chart farts," like when voice recognition turned "psoriasis" into "sorry asses."

Some practices have tried using scribes. But that introduces new employees and new costs, plus the scribe has to be in on private consultations. The other remedy is having lots of pick lists, those screens with little boxes you check to record symptoms or findings.

The EHR designers want to facilitate recording infinite detail, so provide infinite boxes to check. The pain screen asks whether the pain is aching, sharp, burning, or dull; brought on by movement, exertion, deep breathing, acidic foods, or stress.

What's the color/composition/quality/quantity/consistency of the mucus/stool/urine/vaginal discharge/vomitus? And so on, *ad infinitum*. Any slightly OCD provider (and all doctors are obsessive compulsive by necessity) will get lost in space, spending hours trying to check every damn applicable box.

Then some screens are just daft. On the endocrinology screen, there's an option for "clitoral enlargement" (not something I've ever seen or diagnosed in over forty years of practice), but not for hot flashes, which I think every menopausal woman I've ever treated has experienced.

The ENT screen on one system has every kind of tonsillar pathology—bulbus/cryptic/exudative/friable—but there's no option for postnasal drainage, which anyone with a sinus infection or allergies knows about all too well (though possibly only by the technical name, "loogies").

Additionally, the documents EHRs produce are totally out of control. It makes me wonder about the geeks who build computer systems in general. As in any field, it's so easy to generate massive quantities of verbiage, and computer-generated medical documents tend to be quite lengthy and composed of gobbledygook.

Consults from specialists run to six or seven pages, padded with long lists of past medicines, negative findings, all sorts of garbage, and it's virtually impossible to find what the consultant actually thought.

ER reports are the same. They're longwinded, with all sorts of irrelevant information, like what kind of car the patient hit in the motor vehicle accident, but only an unhelpful diagnosis of "leg pain."

Then there's the patient who presents with abdominal pain. After a zillion tests, he has an assessment and diagnosis of "abdominal pain." But there is a code: 789.00—abdominal pain, unspecified—so a bill can be generated, as well as a CYA note for the lawyer saying "Patient was in stable condition and fit for discharge."

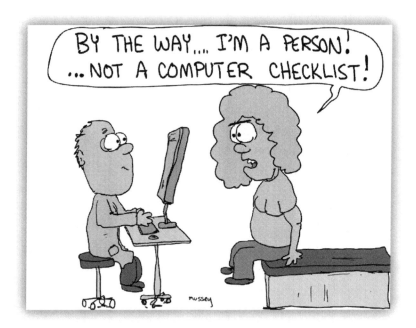

COMPUTERIZED ADVERSITY

Doctors' resistance and incessant complaints aren't just PMS and technophobia, though; they do have some justifications.

For starters, we haven't exactly been given cutting-edge technologies to work with. "Physicians find themselves locked into pre–Internet-era electronic health records," claims a scathing article in the June 2012 *NEJM* by Kenneth D. Mandl, M.D., M.P.H., and Isaac S. Kohane, M.D., Ph.D.

While the rest of the world is enjoying huge improvements in storage, search, communications, graphics, and analysis, "doctors become increasingly bound to documentation and communication products that are functionally decades behind those they use in their 'civilian' life," they say.

"What is also beyond doubt," notes an article in *The New York Times* in June 2011, "is that the promise of digital records will be unfulfilled if doctors refuse to adopt them because they consider the technology cumbersome, time-consuming and possibly dangerous."

Criticizing these hopeless doctors for not getting on board, Maureen Gaffney, chief medical information officer at Winthrop University Hospital in Minneola, New York, said physicians don't necessarily see the potential benefits of electronic records.

"The true benefit is the ability to exchange information in a real-time manner. Physicians can talk in near real time, and have immediate access to test results and lab results. Electronic health records improve communications and will expedite care for the patient," she said.

But I invite her to come visit the Moss Clinic or other locations to find the real truth. All these systems don't talk to each other. Also, some institutions are so worried about security they won't let you access their system, as is the case with the new HCA hospital in my town.

At the clinic, we've given up trying to get access. So, if a patient has been recently discharged from there, we have to wing it until we can get hold of someone to fax us a copy of the report. In the meantime, I have to try to deduce what the cardiologist thought by what medicines he put my patient on, or I have to just hope the follow-up CT scan of the chest didn't show that shadow enlarging. In other words, my patients are getting less than optimal care.

Computers are capable of communicating accurately and quickly enough that I can take money out of my American bank account using an ATM in India. From my U.S. office, I can instantly make a dinner reservation at a restaurant in Madrid and buy train tickets from there to Seville. So why can't I just get this essential medical information?

Much of the blame goes to the fact that there are 700-something competing vendors with about 1,750 distinct products that lack interoperability (i.e., they won't "talk to" each other). The vendors all jealously guard their own systems to "protect their prices and market share," accuse the *NEJM* authors.

Vendors pop up overnight like mushrooms and then go out of business or overhaul their EHR systems. The medical groups using their products suddenly find themselves having to start over again and buy all new software.

And I constantly marvel at the mismatch between what the designers think doctors need and want and what they actually need and want. I can't help but wonder if the manufacturers ever consult a doctor when building an EHR system.

This seems typical of the geeks of the computer world, who seem incapable of understanding how the brains of mere mortals work. Have you ever found *Help* on your computer to be helpful? It always seems to be this massive, incomprihensible overload of information telling you ten different ways to do anything, but without any common-sense guidance. It's ironic for an industry focused on improving communication.

To further editorialize, this whole business of getting the industry of medicine digitized seems a microcosm of the political dysfunction dividing the country and exemplifying the worst of both worlds.

On one hand, you have big government imposing requirements and regulations, which everyone resents. On the other hand, you have private enterprises acting in true entrepreneurial fashion, greedily maximizing profits by refusing to cooperate and do what's best for the public. Maybe the pharmaceutical industry is their role model.

Despite the glitches and the bitching and moaning, EHR holds great promise, though there is one last snafu worth mentioning: EHR means all your eggs are in one basket.

In the satellite office when I worked for Pratt, we were connected to the server in the main office by a single phone line that had a bad habit of losing its connection.

When that happened, we were completely screwed. We couldn't access anything—not the schedule, the charts, the labs, e-mail—and patients got all huffy when they'd been coming in for years but the doctors couldn't remember their names without the chart. When we lost connection, there was this rising hysteria and risk of the doctors either stroking out or throwing things.

So if you happen to be at the doctor's office when suddenly this tense hush falls and all you hear are whispers amongst the staff that "the computers are down," just get out before all hell breaks loose.

ADAPTATION

When your doctor finally installs an EHR system, it will certainly change your interactions. The main thing people complain of is that the doctor pays more attention to the computer than to them, and patients feel a bit like they're interrupting his playing with a new toy.

By necessity, the doctor looks at his computer screen instead of making that all-important eye contact. Though hopefully he'll glance up from time to time.

Out of concern for the dissociating effect of computers on doctor/patient relationships, the profession's spin doctors and gurus of EHR etiquette make suggestions. They tell doctors to at least continue voice communication; explain that you're looking through labs to find the last cholesterol level, for example. Involve the patient more by showing them the list of results on the screen. Maybe you can kindly and gently help train your doctor in good EHR etiquette, too, as he stumbles through adaptation.

SMARTPHONES

A few words about smartphones, which are of course just little mobile computers with the helpful facility of being able to make phone calls, seems in order.

Mobile internet access allows instant acquisition of information. Recently, when at the mall, my daughter called because her friend was flipping out, convinced she had multiple sclerosis (one of the disease hypochondriacs often think they have). After a quick review of the symptoms on WebMD, I could call her right back and allay her friend's anxieties by assuring her the symptoms she described were not consistent with MS.

Having the Epocrates app on my phone, in my pocket at all times, is invaluable when seeing patients. It lets me instantly look up drug doses and other information which my ragged-out brain is incapable of retaining.

Smartphones also facilitate carrying around a lot of information (mine has endless to-do lists, shopping lists, diary notes, etc.). It can even store your personal health record, which you're about to read about.

These mobile devices also increase communication between doctors and patients and support some amazing medical apps to monitor your every bodily function, even detecting sexually transmitted diseases. But I'll get into all this in more detail in *Getting the Right Future.*

YOUR PERSONAL HEALTH RECORDS

Under the umbrella of EHRs are personal health records (PHRs). Your PHR is a collection of all your health records, conveniently gathered together in one file and stored safely in your possesion. This is a compilation of information every patient should assemble, maintain, and bring to their appointments, whether they're with your regular doctor, a specialist, or at a hospital.

Without information about a patient's history, even the smartest doctor in the world has limited ability to help. Patients have this idea that all their medical history, all their prescriptions, every specialist's note, and everything else about them is in their chart.

Wrong.

All that vital information has to be obtained. If you're not completely ga-ga, you can provide some medical history yourself. Still, patients are not always the best historians; they forget, they get longwinded, and sometimes they don't tell you the truth, the whole truth, and nothing but the truth. Or, at their most extreme, as Dr. House is fond of pointing out, patients lie.

Deaf and mute patients present a challenge, though I've had some communicate sufficiently with a creative combination of written notes and miming worthy of Marcel Marceau. It's hard, though, to mime the results of a lab test or what the ENT had to say. The records are important.

Even if you have all your vocal capacities and are a paragon of honesty, your doctor often needs information you don't have. What did the cardiologist think about your irregular heartbeat? What was the pathology of the skin lesion the dermatologist biopsied? What did the MRI of your lumbar spine show?

You'd be amazed (disgusted?) how often this stuff is not in the chart, though this is something computerization should help fix.

If nobody knows whether the spot on your lung was there three years ago and whether it's changed, you're liable to be en route to some knife-happy surgeon. If your doctor doesn't know you always had a weak left arm from a birth injury, you may be in the ER receiving unnecessary clot-buster medicines for a stroke after fainting.

COMPILING YOUR PHR

Compile your own comprehensive PHR, just like the one you always thought your doctor has. This can be challenging. It requires scouring around and getting records from doctors, hospitals, labs, imaging departments, therapists, pharmacies, etc.

Incidentally, as further encouragement to the value of this, your record can be helpful for more than just consulting with medical personnel. When I had to change insurance companies, trying to remember all the medical issues my wife, two daughters, and I had was a nightmare.

Getting your own doctor's records should be relatively easy, though you may encounter resistance and the issue of ownership. Your medical records are in a chart owned by your doctor or the hospital. In the good old days, it was not thought proper for patients to have access to their own charts; if the nurse caught you peeking at your records, it felt like being busted. There's also an element of the doctor and his staff feeling like you don't trust them, and giving you a bit of the cold shoulder as a result.

But the dreaded HIPAA, the mere mention of which strikes fear in to the hearts of doctors) has formalized your right to access your own records. It was passed in 1996, and is seen by many as the epitome of Big Brother, with its threat of punitive censorship for transgressions and its "extensive and confusing" verbiage, as Trisha Torrey puts it.

However, it's good for patients, affirming their right to their medical records (through appropriate request procedures). It also requires your doctor keep them for six years after you leave the practice.

There are grounds for refusing you access. The main one is if the doctor believes letting you see his notes would endanger him. The general idea, though, is that patients have the right to unfettered access.

You can get an informational brochure about HIPAA regulations, spelling out your rights, from the Health and Human Services at www.hhs.gov/ocr/privacy/hipaa/understanding.

It would appear the discomfort doctors and their staff feel about letting patients see their notes is unfounded, judging by the response to the "Open Notes" initiative conducted by the Robert Wood Johnson Foundation, reported in the October 2012 *Annals of Internal Medicine*. It gave a group of patients electronic access to their doctors' notes. Patients didn't get riled up reading what their doctors had written about them. Rather, it was called "a powerful tool in helping improve the lives of patients."

Nor were other fears valid, like that longer, more explicit notes would be needed; that there would be more questions and messages from patients; and that ambiguous abbreviations doctors use, like "SOB" as an abbreviation for "shortness of breath" would be misinterpreted by patients as what doctors thought of them.

Of course, even when you do get free access to your doctor's notes, unless he's computerized, you're still going to have to decipher his chicken scratch.

The VA is in the vanguard. They recently launched the Blue Button program that allows veterans to access or download their entire medical record.

What To Get

A basic PHR should include:

- Records of blood pressure and blood sugars, especially if you are hypertensive or diabetic
- As many lab results as possible, or certainly the most recent, which are generally easily obtained from the lab

- Consultation reports from other doctors, whether in the hospital or as an outpatient
- Hospital records, particularly the discharge summary, copies of studies, consultation reports, and operative reports if you had some procedure
- A family history (go to www.familyhistory.hhs.gov for help), and consider getting your genome sequenced (more on this in *Getting the Right Future*)
- A social history covering exposure to different environments and types of work
- A record of medicines and treatments that have been tried and what happened
- The name and contact of all your doctors and details of your insurance policy

PHR COMPANIES

As you might expect, there are companies who see helping people compile their PHR as a business opportunity. A few I came across are:

Zweena Health (www.zweenahealth.com), which gathers your information from your doctor, converts it to digital form, and creates a personal record accessible to you, chosen friends and family, and your doctor. "Doctors trust Zweena information because it comes from the health records stored in their offices," notes the website. The company also claims to provide information to help make proactive healthcare decisions.

They charge a monthly access fee of $10, then $85 for twenty pages of digitalized records (the amount they recommend for a single person's PHR). They charge more if you have more people, obviously.

MyMediConnect (www.mymediconnect.net) is a similar company. It recently absorbed the popular company PassportMD. They claim superiority by offering "medical reminder messages, to securely communicate with your doctor, track your health and fitness," and provide "trusted answers to all medical questions."

Microsoft Health Vault (www.healthvault.com) also collects health information. It says you can "be better prepared for doctor visits and unexpected emergencies," by creating a more complete picture of your health, and it says it can help you achieve your fitness goals.

As I say, I came across these options, but I'm not necessarily recommending them. *InformationWeek* published a fairly comprehensive review of "9 Popular Personal Health Record Tools" by Anthony Vecchione on April 16, 2012.

If you're going to use such a service, the Nationwide Health Information Network (www.healthIT.gov) provides standards and policies to help you know what safeguards you need to "enable secure exchange of information over the internet." Take a look.

Keeping It All

Having pulled together all your information, you then have to decide how to store it. In some musty paper file in a closet like mine? The new way is in cyberspace, or the cloud, though as noted, some people have concerns about hackers getting access to their medical information.

It's now feasible to have your PHR stored digitally on something like a credit card. When you're run over by a bus and carted off to the ER, you can whip out your Visa or Mastercard and your entire medical history.

The Care Medical History Card (medicalhistorybracelet. com/care-medical-history-card/), for example, is available for $39.99 (as is a bracelet alternative). It incorporates a USB thumb drive with plenty of space to store your and/or your family members' medical information. The whole thing is pretty user friendly.

The military uses new-age "dog-tags," or more properly, personal information carriers (PICs). They're thumb drives with high storage capacity. There's even a suggestion that every soldier have a whole body CT scan stored digitally on the PIC so when they're blown apart, there will be a baseline to know what they looked like beforehand.

Radio frequency identification (RFID) chips are even more space age.

An RFID was credited with saving the life of William Koretsky, a 44-year-old sergeant with the Bergen County Police Department. In May 2006, he crashed his car into a tree during a high-speed chase. He was taken to the hospital, where an ER scan revealed an RFID chip in his arm that had been implanted in 2004 for identification purposes at the suggestion of his police chief. Doctors retrieved the ID number, identified Koretsky using an online database, reviewed his health history, and learned that he had type 1 diabetes. It was a crucial piece of information, which, if unknown, could have meant the condition went untreated and been the end of him regardless of his injuries.

"I was unable to communicate, but the chip talked for me," Koretsky is reported as saying on The European Molecular Biology Organization website.

The public's "embrace of PHR is notably weak," says Topol in *The Creative Destruction of Medicine.* Despite a "clear rationale for their potential benefit," only 2.7 percent of patients have assembled a PHR, he reports. According to an American Medical Association survey, only 44 percent of doctors are willing to use a patient's PHR as part of their efforts.

I wonder if this luke-warm embrace by doctors—and the subliminal implication that a patient is hostile or distrustful if they ask for a copy of their records—isn't some resistance to the idea of patients getting more involved and empowered.

CHAPTER 4

GETTING THE RIGHT TREATMENT

———◆———

APPROACH WITH CAUTION

TREATMENT IS THE ALL-IMPORTANT CULMINATION, the endpoint after you've found the right doctor, achieved the right diagnosis, and gathered the right information. Next comes the serious decision about what treatment is right for you. Pills? Surgery? A shot? Physical therapy? Talk therapy? Diet? Exercise? Alternative therapy? The possibilities are practically endless.

Note that a good number of treatments once hailed as the best thing since sliced bread have undergone not "course corrections," says Steven Kussin, M.D., but "neck-snapping 180-degree hairpin turns."

Bleeding and purging were popular treatments, no matter that the patient was in circulatory collapse from bloodloss, dehydration, or toxic shock. George Washington was relieved of the equivalent of eight units of blood for a throat infection, which he then promptly died from. Mercury was considered a great medicine, especially for syphilis, and radium a superb tonic, until both were found to be extremely toxic.

More recently, aspirin was touted to prevent heart attacks, ACE inhibitors were claimed to reduce mortality before cardiac bypass surgery, and bisphosphonates were good for osteoporosis—and then not. Hormone replacement therapy (HRT), echinacea, saturated fats, eggs, and breast self exams have all been recipients of recent radical changes of heart.

Then, a number of medicines get pulled from the shelves when after-marketing surveillance shows them to cause some previously undetected diabolical side effect.

The wise practitioner (and patient) lets someone else be the guinea pig, waiting until any new treatment—medicines in particular—have been in use for a while.

A WORD ON TERMINOLOGY

Before we get started, let me comment on the difference between "medicines" and "medications."

There is none, of course, except that "medicines" is shorter and more concise. Using "medicines" conflicts with the American imperative of utilizing—er, using—a longer word when a shorter one would do.

In England, the person who administers dangerous sedatives (a pinch at a time, like a gourmet chef) and holds you in that suspended animation between life and death, protecting you as best he can from the surgeon, is an "anesthetist." In America, an anesthetist is a mere nurse. The doctor is altogether grander, so has the more cumbersome title of "anesthesiologist."

But preferring my simple, English ways, I'll stick to "medicines."

Also, as you probably know, every drug has at least two names. Manufacturers give their medicines catchy, friendly-sounding, easy-to-remember brand names. But each drug has a generic name, identified as the "active ingredient."

My cousin Ron, a medicinal chemist, claims generic names are long and difficult to discourage generic prescribing. If you have arthritis, but also a sensitive stomach, and your doctor wants to put you on the generic for Arthrotec, he has to write "diclofenac/misoprostol." If he wants to stop your blood from clotting with generic Plavix, he has to try to spell "clopidogrel." Though in fairness, these days he can usually write the brand name he's so familiar with and check the "substitution permissible" box.

DRUGS, DRUGS, DRUGS

Taking some kind of medicine is the most common form of treatment in our drug-preponderent culture, whether administered as pills, shots, suppositories, pessaries, lozenges, or applied to some part or another as liquids, creams, ointments, linements, or lotions.

We are a drug-addicted culture. In any given week, more than four in five U.S. adults take at least one medicine and almost one-third take at least five, according to the Institute of Medicine. And 90 percent of seniors take some kind of medicine. In *Our Daily Meds: How the Pharmaceutical Companies Transformed Themselves into Slick Marketing Machines and Hooked the Nation on Prescription Drugs*, journalist Melody Petersen notes that most seniors in the U.S. today take two to three times more medicines than they need.

The trend is getting worse, too; there were more medicines taken in one day in 2005 than in one month in 1950. The industry pulls in up to $300 billion per year.

Our addiction is born of sloth, to a large extent. Egged on by a massively profitable and manipulative industry that's all too happy with the attitude of "screw the diet/exercise/deprivation/ self control... just give me a pill" for whatever ails.

One of my standard (bad) jokes is that we never get detailed by company reps selling diets or exercise machines, despite the Diabetes Prevention Program study showing that diet and exercise is better than the most commonly used diabetes drug, metformin.

I consider myself somewhat pharmacophobic, and I consider having to take medicine for anything a bit of a failure. I've always tried to practice by the maxim "the less medicines, the better."

I've also always been wary of the fandanglings of the pharmaceutical industry, but I had no idea just how pervasive and insidious a problem it is until I started researching for this book.

Now I'm horrified at how much of a sucker I've been to the industry's manipulations, at how much I've been misled by their wicked ways. I'm left wondering how many of my patients I prescribed more expensive or less effective drugs for lack of due diligence in seeking out the objective truth. And I wonder how many of my colleagues are in the same boat and how many still innocently stumble along, oblivious, not aware enough about the situation.

I realize it's often necessary to take medicines to stay alive or alleviate discomfort, particularly because we're so bad at lifestyle modifications and practicing prevention. So, grudgingly I prescribe them.

The hoodwinked doctor does the drug company's bidding at the office visit. Consider how it typically goes: You spend a long time sitting in the waiting room, listlessly thumbing through dogeared, out-of-date *National Geographic* issues before the nurse takes you back.

Then you wait for the doctor in the exam room, reading for the umpteenth time all those friendly notices that adorn the walls, like, "We don't bill for co-payments" and "The doctor can only address one problem per visit."

Finally, the door opens and a middle-aged, slightly breathless, slightly disheveled doctor in a slightly too tight, immaculately starched, buttoned up white lab coat, button down collar, and tie with silkscreen picture of his kids enters. He sits on the rolling stool, stabs his finger at a number on a paper in the chart and says, "Well John, I think it's time to put you on some blood pressure pills."

You have some misgiving that your pressure was high this morning because it was already 43 minutes after your appointment time when the nurse called you back and checked it. But the doctor looks busy. This is a straightforward problem. Everyone's told you what a great guy he is (which is presumably why he's so busy and so late), so you don't question him.

As you come out of the exam room, he calls to his nurse, "Cathy, find John here some Benicar. Give him a couple of weeks' worth please." Then, as he stands with his hand on the door handle of the next exam room, looking at the next chart, says, "So, John, come back in a couple of weeks for a blood pressure check."

As you wait like a spare part for your samples, you notice a rather attractive blonde woman bent forward, emphasizing her cleavage, checking boxes of medicines in the drug closet. As she straightens up, you notice a nametag with the Benicar logo pinned to her ample bosom.

By now, the doctor has come out of the other room and walks over to the drug closet saying, "Hey Shannon, you're looking good, how are you? Any coffee this morning?" She smiles broadly, smoothes her blouse, and points to a Starbucks travel pack and cups on the countertop.

The doctor, leering, ambles over and pours himself a cup. Staring very obviously at her cleavage, he starts telling her how he's been prescribing a lot of Benicar, how much he enjoyed the drug dinner, and that she should come out on his boat some time.

Meanwhile, you shuffle out of the office clutching your brown paper bag of samples like some party favor, thinking, "I guess I've got high blood pressure. But thank god I have a great doctor who knows which is the best medicine for it."

TRYING DRUG TRIALS

It's a long road to get a medicine to market.

It all starts with identifying a need, though the "need" is often relative. Most medicines are developed for illnesses that already have treatments; diseases without treatments are rarities.

"Most new drugs and new indications for older drugs do not represent any significant therapeutic advance." They don't "add to the clinical possibilities," says Donald W. Light from the Program in Human Biology at Stanford University and Rebecca Warburton from the University of Medicine and Dentistry of New Jersey. Only a measly 0.2 percent of new products are any kind of "major innovation where no treatment was previously available," they note.

The new medicine usually has only a marginal advantage, if any, over what's already available. Maybe it has a better delivery system so you don't have to take it so frequently or it's a little "cleaner," with fewer side effects.

In *The Truth About Drug Companies*, former editor of *The New England Journal of Medicine* Marcia Angell notes from 1998 to 2002, 77 percent of new drugs were classified by the FDA as being "no better than the drugs already on the market to treat the same condition."

The term in the profession is "me-too" drugs, as companies try to get on some lucrative bandwagon like high cholesterol, high blood pressure, diabetes, or depression—conditions for which people take expensive medicines for the rest of their lives.

And you were wondering why there are so many blood pressure medicines.

If the company has been able to concoct some slight unique twist to a molecule, they can secure a twenty-year patent, prohibiting any generic equivalent until it expires.

This requires armies of chemistry nerds tinkering with a whole mess of different chemicals, trying to hit on the exact right side chains, radical, or carbon ring, whatever key fits the lock on the appropriate receptor site of the cells to bring down your blood pressure, lower your cholesterol, reduce your stomach acid, lift your depression, open your airways, give you a usable erection, or whatever.

This potential new chemical is first tested on animals, usually those long-suffering lab rats. Then, assuming it did something useful and the rats didn't all die, a "clinical trial" is performed on human lab rats. The effect on humans tells if the medicine is going to be something useful and, very importantly, if it has any serious adverse effects.

Detecting adverse effects is not an infallible process. A string of drugs (Trovan, Fen-Phen, Raxar, Posicor, Vioxx, Propulsid, Zelnorm, Rezulin, Lotronox, Pemoline, Dexatrim, Baycol, etc.) have been withdrawn after release when a seriously harmful effect came to light in post-market surveillance.

An article in a 2009 *Archives of Internal Medicine* talks about the "seven year rule." Cautious doctors wait until a drug has been on the market for seven years before prescribing it because of the dangers of adverse effects that didn't manifest before a license was granted.

The FDA requires that drug trials be multi-centered (information must be gathered from several different locations), show superiority to a placebo (be more effective than an inactive "sugar pill," but not that it's more effective than anything else already on the market), and be double blind (neither the patients nor the doctors know who's getting the placebo or the medicine). This is a long process of testing on a lot of subjects, which makes it expensive.

Nowadays, drug companies, rather than academic centers, nearly always sponsor clinical trials. Starting under Regan's administration, a seriese of moves by Congress—most significantly the Bayh-Dole Act—allowed tax-sponsored organizations like the NIH to patent discoveries formerly left to the public domain and enter deals with pharmaceutical companies, notes Angell.

Since then, an unhealthy trend has emerged for trials to be performed by private companies. In 1990, 80 percent of trials were done by academic institutions; within a decade, it was less than 40 percent. Today, as Angell puts it, researchers are "little more than hired hands."

Industry-sponsored research is four times more likely to produce a favorable result for the sponsoring company's product. And unfortunately, only large companies have the bankroll to spend the $1.2 billion claimed to be the cost of bringing a drug to market.

This whopping sum is used to justify the high price of medicines, but plenty of skeptics maintian this figure is overblown.

In the Febuary 7, 2011 *BioSocieties* online publication, two researchers allege drug companies obfuscate the numbers, which are in reality far lower. They also knock the companies for claiming drugs are more beneficial than they are. They also question the time it takes, saying it's only half what the industry claims. And they make the point that much of the research drug companies capitalize on is done through tax-funded organizations like the NIH.

Angell talks about research and development costs for the top ten companies being somewhere between only 11 and 14 percent of profits. In contrast, "a staggering 36 percent of sales revenue" went to "marketing and administration." She also mentions how the new FDA commissioner, Dr. Mark McClellan, "seemed to swallow hook, line, and sinker the fiction that drug prices have to be high to cover research and development costs."

It's true the costs of bringing a drug to market (especially stage 3 testing on humans) is steadily becoming more expensive. But the hope is genomics and tissue culture techniques will bring the costs down again, but more on that in *Getting the Right Future.*

This business of drug companies—and not the investigators—sponsoring and having ownership of the clinical trials is undesirable, says Roy. M. Poses, M.D., president of the Foundation for Integrity and Responsibility in Medicine. He claims it allows "the sponsor, but not the investigator, to alter study design" and pull fandangles like inadequately blinding the investigators, giving the drug to innapropriate age groups, and giving innapropriate doses.

They can also withold information that doesn't look good (e.g., only the favorable first six months of data from a year-long Celebrex trial to assess heart attack risk was released by the manufacturer) or pick a spurious endpoint (for example, there's a critical distinction between lowering cholesterol levels and reducing heart attacks and coronary artery disease, the true goal of cholesterol-lowering medicines).

The sponsor has control over the statistical analysis, which can be manipulated in plenty of ways that have real bearings on how good or bad a medicine looks. It brings to mind something Benjamin Disraeli said about "lies, damn lies, and statistics."

Like many doctors, I'm no statistician, and certainly not savvy enough to pick apart the statistics the drug companies offer as persuasive evidence of how wonderful their products are. So I was interested in the *Business Week* article sent to me by an old school chum on treatment for high cholesterol. It's from 2008, following the fracas about the ENHANCE trial of a new Schering-Plough cholesterol-lowering medicine, Vytorin, which appeared to show no superiority over good old-fashioned Zocor.

Business Week talked about another cholesterol-lowering medicine, the blockbuster Pfizer product Lipitor, that had netted the company $12.4 billion in 2008. Pfizer was claiming Lipitor "reduces the heart attack rate by 36 percent" in people with multiple risk factors. It sounds impressive, and that's how they were convincing doctors.

But as the statisticians at *Business Week* pointed out, if you look more carefully, what the numbers show is that over the forty-month course of the trial, 3 percent of patients taking placebo had heart attacks versus 2 percent taking Lipitor.

Yes, it amounted to about a one-third difference in the number of heart attacks. But looked at another way, it's a 1 percent difference between the two groups. So, 100 people had to take Lipitor for more than three years for one to be protected from a heart attack, and the other ninety-nine gained no benefit, risked side effects and, in the real world, would've had the cost, too.

This is the number needed to treat (NNT) discussed in *Getting the Right Diagnosis*. It can give a very different feel to a drug and have significant weight with doctors' willingness to prescribe. Many experts promote the NNT as the most important statistic. In the above case, the NNT is 100; 100 people had to be treated for one to benefit.

The *Business Week* article gained notoriety in the drug industry. When I made reference to it to the Pfizer rep at the time, she changed from charm and coquettishness to pouting and made some snide remark about "oh *that* article."

I hate to say it, but even British pharmaceutical companies are devious and attempt to take advantage of the power that comes with ownership of drug trials. Boots Pharmaceuticals tried to suppress publication of the results of a study it commissioned to show its thyroid supplement Synthroid had superior "bioequiva-lence" over generics.

Unfortunately, researcher Betty Dong from the University of California in San Francisco didn't find this to be the case. She noted the cheaper drugs were virtually interchangeable and using them instead of Synthroid could reduce health care costs by $365 million per year.

This did not please Boots.

Although this study had been accepted for publication in the prestigious *Journal of the American Medical Association*, Boots, which happened to be in the middle of negotiations to sell its drug division to German company BASF for $1.4 billion, suddenly claimed the study was flawed and tried to invoke a sneaky clause in the contract saying the paper couldn't be published without its consent.

Boots came up with another study showing Synthroid was superior. It was published in the somewhat obscure *American Journal of Therapeutics*. By an amazing coincidence, Dr. Gilbert Mayor, director of Medical Services for Boots, just happened to be an editor of the publication.

Apart from these obvious fandangles of owning the study, there is also a nebulous, somewhat inexplicable benefit. A study conducted by the University of California, San Francisco looked at the sponsorship of some 200 clinical trials comparing one cholesterol medicine against a competitor. Though no exact reason could be pinpointed, it showed a study of a given drug was thrity-five times more likely to favor the sponsoring company's product over the competitor.

As I say, drug companies are about the only ones who can afford to sponsor trials. But this is such standard practice now, I think doctors don't give a second thought to the idea that sponsorship could have some bearing on the outcome.

The journals do have a disclaimer about sponsorship at the end of studies, but in print so small you need a magnifying glass.

Ownership of the study also facilitates suppression of the numbers you don't like. The FDA requires two studies that show the drug is more effective than a placebo, but it doesn't matter how many trials are done that *don't* show this. These don't have to be published; they can just be discreetly buried.

PRESTIGIOUS PUBLICATION PERVERSITIES

Successfully completed trials are written up and submitted to some learned journal for publication. The best known are the *Journal of the American Medical Association (JAMA)* and *New England Journal of Medicine (NEJM)*. There are zillions, though, with each specialty usually having its own organization or society with its own arcane, esoteric journal, like *The Journal of Pediatric Endocrinology and Metabolism* or *Electroencephalography and Neurophysiology*. Good for some light reading.

So, there are almost endless journals to submit your study to. The good ones are "peer reviewed," meaning a panel of experts in the relevant field looks at the study and decides if it's of sufficient quality and interest to warrant acceptance.

But the idea that journals are unimpeachable sources of objective information on drugs has a few pitfalls.

In *Doctor, Your Patient Will See You Now*, Kussin quotes respected epidemiologist John Loannidis saying that drug companies sponsoring trials "has taken away the reassurance that study designs are sound, properly conducted and that its results are properly interpreted." In 2009, the online medical journal *PLOS Medicine* noted that medical journals "may increasingly become closer to works of fiction, telling stories dictated by variouse lobbyists, than works of science."

Ghostwriting is threatening the validity of the journals. This is when ready-made scientific articles are placed in leading medical journals, "carrying the imprimatur of influential academic leaders," claims personal injury lawyer Alexander Shunnarah on his website. Some top university scientist reviews them and assigns his or her name to them, then they're sent to some learned journal as an original paper.

In its campaign to promote the slimming pill Redux, Wyeth-Ayerst paid $180,000 to the medical publishing company Excerpta Medica to churn out articles. Wyeth again used ghostwriters in its campaign to counteract reports on the apparent risk of their hormone replacement therapy, Prempro. Claims were made that Prempro was causing breast cancer and vascular disease. Wyeth is reported to have used the company Design Write to produce more than fifty articles for peer-reviewed publications.

Another pitfall of this dependence on learned journals is that it prompts counterfeits.

Grasping an opportunity, the large and (formerly) prestigious medical publishing company Elsevier (publisher of that supposedly inviolable British journal, *The Lancet*) sullied its reputation by publishing the *Australasian Journal of Bone and Joint Medicine*. It looked just like—and masqueraded as—a respectable peer-reviewed journal.

But in reality, it was "a collection of reprinted articles," some ghostwritten and paid for by Merck, which "lavished unalloyed praise on Merck drugs," according to Harriet Washington, fellow in medical ethics at Harvard Medical School and author of *Deadly Monopolies: The Shocking Corporate Takeover of Life Itself—And the Consequences for Our Health and Our Medical Future.*

There appeared to be a total of fifty of these "Big Pharma advertisements passed off as medical publications," according to "forensic librarian" Jonathan Rochkind. He claimed Elsevier, this former "queen" of the medical publishing field, should now be considered a "high-priced call girl."

Even real journals with papers written by real researchers are suspect. "All journals are bought—or cleverly used—by the pharmaceutical industry," laments Richard Smith, former editor of the *British Medical Journal* (U.K. equivalent of *JAMA*).

In part, they are overwhelmed by advertising. Many of these journals "carried more advertising than editorial pages," writes Washington. Many of the most prestigious journals carry "glossy, full-color inserts that were longer than the journals' longest articles," she says.

The advertisements in these journals provide up to 99 percent of their revenue and are their very lifeblood, to the point where journals advertise for advertisers. *JAMA* touts its "priceless audience at a price you can afford."

It's not just the quantity of ads, however. The FDA has had to come up with guidelines for advertisers, with the outrageous requirement that ads have "true statements relating to side effects, contraindications, and effectiveness" and a "fair and balanced statement" about risks and benefits.

Indicative of the pharmaceutical industry's "enthusiasm" is that the FDA had to issue eighty-eight letters of reprimand.

The *Annals of Internal Medicine* performed an analysis of the advertisements in its own pages to see how well they adhered to the guidelines. The reviewers determined 40 percent of pharmaceutical ads failed the "fair and balanced" test and 44 percent would lead to improper prescribing.

When it published these results, the drug companies got huffy and withdrew their $1.5 million in advertising. Those righteous editors had to resign "to save the journal." Coeditor Robert Fletcher commented that if you ever wonder if the drug companies "play hardball, that was a pretty good demonstration that they do."

Since then, a new group has taken over. It's a more deferential bunch, it would seem by their care in inviting commentary before publishing an editorial on high drug prices. And the advertising is back.

Like all consumers, doctors tend to maintain a healthy skepticism about advertising, even of drugs. But doctors expect that editorial content—especially in a publication like *NEJM*—will not be promotional. They presume it to be beyond pharmaceutical company influence, unsullied, unbiased, and true.

Dream on.

The Redux story is a good example of how the long, pervasive fingers of pharmaceutical influence find their way into every pie. And, since Redux is an appetite suppressant, pie is an appropriate metaphor.

The drug's generic ingredient is dexfenfluramine, an ingredient in another slimming pill, Fen-Phen.

Redux came out in 1996 and immediately became a wild success, enthusiastically embraced by those in the pill culture who were having trouble losing weight with the whole will power thing.

Soon reports were surfacing from Europe of fenfluramine users developing primary pulmonary hypertension, a nasty disease that causes high blood pressure in your lungs that can cause irreversible and severe shortness of breath. There were also reports of heart valve damage with Fen-Phen.

In the middle of this, *NEJM* published an editorial by Jo Ann Mason, M.D., Dr.P.H., of Harvard Medical School and Gerald A. Faich, M.D., M.P.H., an epidemiologist from University of Pennsylvania and former FDA official, who had done research on Redux.

This editorial defended Redux, claiming the risk of pulmonary hypertension was "small and appears to be outweighed by benefits when the drug is used appropriately."

With such a ringing endorsement from such a respected source, the drug's reputation—and sales—received a significant boost. But soon after publication, it became apparent that the two had financial ties to the manufacturer. They had been paid by Wyeth-Ayerst and other companies involved in manufacture to give evidence at an FDA hearing supporting Redux. The month the editorial was published, Faich had acted as a consultant for the company in their European operation. In addition, Wyeth-Ayers had paid $180,000 for nine ghostwritten articles published in various journals.

The *NEJM* editors considered this a violation of their prohibition on writings from sources with "regular" and "ongoing" financial ties and later issued an apology for the editorial. Shortly after, the FDA concluded the benefits of Redux did not out weigh the risks and it got pulled from the market.

The salient point is, of course, that a journal as prestigious and reputable as *NEJM* couldn't avoid contributors in the pay of the industry.

Maybe it's an unrealistic idea that we can avoid drug company money and influence in medical journals and other places.

"Ninety-five percent of academic-medicine specialists who assess patented treatments have relationships with pharmaceutical companies," Washington notes. And, somewhat plaintively, in 1992, *NEJM* announced it "gave up its search for objective reviewers." The editors "could find no reviewers that did not accept industry funds," she reports.

Angell says of her time at *NEJM*, "I saw companies exercise a level of control over the way in which research was done which was unheard of when I first came to the journal, and the aim was clearly to load the dice to make sure their drugs looked good."

When drug trials are published in journals, we doctors assiduously read them and put everyone on the new miracle drug because the numbers have been crunched so effectively that it looks brilliant.

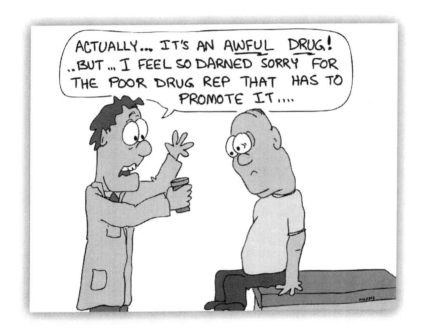

MORE DRUG COMPANY TENTACLES

As noted in *Getting the Right Information*, there are so many arcane, hard-to-digest papers published, it's not practical for doctors to get their information from journals. Just trying to keep up with the basics like the *American Academy of Family Physicians Journal*, *JAMA*, and *NEJM* is too much.

Instead we busy doctors rely on pre-digested information from all sorts of outlets, like drug reps, medical newspapers, computer programs, even cell phone apps these days, and lots of quasi-promotional "education" provided by "thought leaders."

These so-called thought leaders are local or national specialists who speak at meetings, "grand rounds"(a kind of case discussion format hospitals often host), drug dinners, continuing medical education conferences, and the like.

They are often big-name doctors doing research sponsored by drug companies, or they receive a stipend or payment from a company. One cannot help but suspect their opinions of the products are influenced by that relationship.

The companies that sponsor meetings work hard to ensure only the right message gets conveyed. "Drug companies hire doctors to give lectures, but require them to show only the slides that have been approved by the company," complains J. Douglas Bremner, M.D., a professor of psychiatry and radiology at Emory University and author of *Before You Take that Pill.*

It's a practice he's fallen foul of. "I fought not to use company-approved slides and was dropped as a speaker," he says.

Pharmaceutical companies get their feet in the door at medical schools to catch the docs when they're young and impressionable. It seems to be working, judging by reports that 90 percent of medical students have already established a relationship with a drug company by receiving some form of educational material from them, the *Public Library of Science* tells us.

And there are relationships with faculty members and departments of medical schools. Harvard Medical School's dean received $500,000 in research grants since 2007 from Bristol-Myers Squibb. When disclosure was made obligatory, one professor reported an affiliation with forty-seven companies. In

2008, the school as a whole received $8.6 million for basic science research and $3 million for continuing education from the pharmaceutical industry.

Some claim this is innocent, even necessary because medical schools need the money. But too many schools have struck a "Faustian bargain," according to Angell, who's also a Harvard faculty member. She says, "Industry profit motives do not correspond to the scientific aims of academic medicine," and the financing needs to be banned.

Of course, it's that one great commodit—money—that allows drug companies to weild such influence.

The amounts they spend are certainly enough for "thought leaders" to think twice about biting the hand that feeds them. Glendale Press in Glendale, California reports that "eight drug companies have paid doctors across the country more than $320 million since 2009" and "topping the list locally was David Tonnemacher, a Glendale cardiologist who received $114,000 from GlaxoSmithKline."

Doctors, departments, institutions, research projects, and the like that receive sponsorship from drug companies "may tend to favor their product," warns Poses.

A large proportion of decisions made by experts, which we peons follow slavishly, have "no or minimal data" to support them, claims Eric Topol in *The Creative Destruction of Medicine*.

Kussin calls this reliance on thought leaders "emminence-based medicine," as opposed to evidence-based medicine.

MORE DRUG COMPANY DEVIOUSNESS

Some pharmaceutical companies like to push non-FDA-sanctioned ("off-label") uses for drugs and offer good old-fashioned bribes to get doctors to prescribe their products.

The New York Times in September 2009 reported the story of a civil lawsuit against the pharmaceutical company Forest claiming it "illegally marketed both Lexapro and a closely related antidepressant, Celexa, for use in children and paid kickbacks to doctors to induce them to prescribe the medicines." These drugs weren't approved for use in children.

Also in 2009, Eli Lilly agreed to pay $1.4 billion in criminal penalties and settlements in four civil lawsuits when the company was accused of pushing their blockbuster anti-psychotic, Zyprexa, in nursing homes and assisted living facilities.

In November 2013, in what the Department of Justice called "one of the largest healthcare fraud settlements in U.S. history," Johnson and Johnson and its subsidiaries paid more than $2.2 billion to resolve criminal and civil charges over aggressive drug marketing. "The corporation also allegedly paid kickbacks to physicians and to Omnicare—the nation's largest long-term care pharmacy provider," reports the July-August 2014 issue of *AARP Bulletin.*

Just these few examples are a rather disheartening litany, and they don't reflect too well on the drug companies. But the problem's not confined to drugs alone.

Some doctors get kickbacks from medical device manufacturers. Assistant inspector general at the Department of Health and Human Services, Gregory Demske, told a Senate committee in 2008 that "Physicians routinely receive substantial compensation from medical device companies through stock options, royalty agreements, consulting agreements, research grants, and fellowships."

And, then-U.S. Attorney for the District of New Jersey Chris Christie complained, "Many orthopedic surgeons in this country made decisions predicated on how much money they could make, choosing which device to implant by going to the highest bidder."

In 2008, *The New York Times* reported on five leading medical device companies (Stryker, Biomet, DePuy Orthopedics, Smith and Nephew, and Zimmer Holdings) that agreed to pay $310 million in fines to settle civil charges of improper payments to doctors.

Some doctors say it's all legit. They claim to be an essential part of the development process and that relationships with manufacturers are necessary. For example, Dr. Thomas Coon, a surgeon in Red Bluff, California and pioneer of minimally invasive knee surgery told *The New York Times* the broad reach of the government's action had "thrown up in the air" hundreds of company-surgeon relationships. "Who knows how it will come out?" mused Coon.

He declined to reveal how much he was paid by Zimmer Holdings, which halted payments under threat of prosecution. However, Zimmer's records showed Coon was paid $158,420 one year, with an additional $1,944 for air travel, $2,498 for lodgings, $1,034 for meals, $440 for ground transportation, and $10 for a gift. Must have been some gift.

In September 2011, "journalism in the public interest" website ProPublica reported at least fifteen drug and medical device companies have paid $6.5 billion since 2008 to settle accusations of marketing fraud or kickbacks.

Obviously, it's not ideal for your doctor to prescribe a medicine because he's getting kickbacks, rather than because it's what's best for you, or for your surgeon to simply choose the most profitable prosthesis.

In her book *The Empowered Patient*, CNN senior medical correspondent Elizabeth Cohen describes the case of a woman who had agreed to go along with her orthopedic surgeon's recommendation to have a particular artificial disc put in to treat her back pain. It was a disaster, and "I couldn't take enough drugs for the pain," the woman relates.

Only after did she learn her surgeon had accepted thousands of dollars from the manufacturer of the disc. But this is "miniscule compared with the $8 million two other physicians received from this company—each," she writes.

Hopefully the Affordable Care Act's "Sunshine Act" will improve things. It mandates publicizing drug company payments to doctors. To find out if your doctor receives any kind of payments, check at projects.propublica.org/docdollars. As for medical devices, you'll have to ask your doctor if he has any relationships with manufacturers.

Be skeptical if you learn of any relationships, and consider a second opinion on the recommendations your doctor makes.

Another place pharmaceutical companies apparently manage to steer doctors is in the popular drug information program Epocrates.

As noted in *Getting the Right Information*, the conventional source of drug information, the *Physicians' Desk Reference*, is a hideously unwieldy, impractical tome. Epocrates, available online and as a smartphone app, is a real boon. More than 80 percent of physician smartphone owners used it twelve times per weeks, on average, according to Epocrates.

If your doctor takes out his phone in the middle of your consultation and starts pecking away, it doesn't necessarily mean he's texting that nurse on the urology floor he was joking with about sperm samples, or that he's playing Angry Birds; he may be looking up drug information, marveling that he can get the basic version for free.

Or so he thinks.

You wouldn't expect a site used by 50 percent of doctors to be a magnet to drug companies, would you? Especially when more and more doctors are finding themselves too busy to see reps...

The Trojan horse here is called DocAlerts. These alerts transmit "key pharma studies or journal articles" which the website Gaia Health Information and other cynics claim are just thinly disguised promotions. They also point out the overly cozy relationship between Epocrates and the pharmaceutical industry, with current CEO Rosemary A. Crane being an ex-employee of drug companies Johnson and Johnson and Bristol-Myer Squibb.

BIG PHARMA AND THE FDA: A SCARY RELATIONSHIP

The overly cozy and influential relationship between the pharmaceutical industry and the FDA is even more worrisome. The FDA is supposed to regulate the industry in the best interest of the public.

This troubling relationship is largely attributed to the 1992 Prescription Drug User Fee Act. It allowed the chronically understaffed and underfunded FDA to start charging companies for each new drug application it processed.

New drug application fees went up from $100,000 in 1993 to $1.5 million in 2010. Much of this goes toward speeding up the drug approval process, but at the expense of safety, accuses Angell. After a decade of the act, "a record thirteen drugs have had to be withdrawn from the market," she points out.

It effectively means drug companies pay FDA staff salaries. "The FDA started looking upon the industry as their client," charges Sidney Wolfe, M.D., director of Public Citizen's Health Research Group.

Also, there's been a lot of career interplay, with FDA officials sometimes moving to high-paying jobs at pharmaceutical companies, creating the desire to stay on amicable terms. Also, most doctors making up FDA advisory panels receive payments as consultants or get research grants from drug companies.

There are accusations in the March 17, 2005 online edition of *NEJM* about FDA supervisors stifling junior staff wanting to publish data on adverse effects of antidepressents in adolescents and about the osteoporosis medicine Fosamax.

But the most extreme seems to be what was described as "the greatest drug safety catastrophe ... in the history of the world."

Vioxx, made by Merck, was one of two Cox-2 inhibitor anti-inflamatory/arthritis medicines (the other was Celebrex) enjoying great success and sales around 1999. Both significantly reduced the risk of gastrointestinal irritation and bleeding compared with conventional arthritis medicines like ibuprofen and naproxen.

David J. Graham, M.D., M.P.H., associate director of Drug Safety at the FDA, started to have concerns about vascular effects of these medicines. He arranged a study he claimed showed people taking Vioxx had an increased risk of heart attack, 30 to 40 percent of which were fatal.

But Graham's supervisor accused him of performing "junk science," of spreading "scientific rumor," and of prejudice against Merck. He told Graham he could only present the results if he amended his conclusions, which he did "because I thought if I didn't, there was no way that the data would see the light of day."

The FDA contacted the journals the original Vioxx study had already been sent to and tried to stop publication. They threatened Graham with disciplinary action and to "exile him from drug safety work," according to the Government Accountability Project, to which he turned for help.

This saga grabbed media attention when Graham testified at a Congressional hearing about Vioxx. He dramatically announced, "Today we are faced with what may be the single greatest drug safety catastrophe in this country or in the history of the world." He accused the FDA of letting the American people down and betraying the public trust.

It all seems to imply the FDA is more concerned about staying in favor with the industry that is now its paymaster than it is about being a good watchdog.

MINIONS, AKA DRUG REPS

The most direct—and I imagine most effective—drug promotion to doctors is one-on-one coercion by drug reps.

There is one drug rep for every six docs, providing "food, flattery, and friendship to create reciprocity," as Angell puts it. The Pew Trust says the industry spends somewhere between $20 billion and $57 billion per year on this army. Some soldiers are "hail-fellow-well-met," square-jawed, assertive men in blazers and power ties. But more and more these days, reps are young, attractive, buxom babes with that irresistible, come-hither manner (is this something they're taught in training?).

The New York Times reports in "Gimmie an Rx! Cheerleaders Pump Up Drug Sales" that the industry has found a ready source of, if not well-informed candidates, commodities that get the doctor's attention for a couple of minutes (if he happens to be a man).

They come to detail us about the latest—and therefore usually most expensive—products, with glossy color brochures showing bar graphs and pie charts. They're studies in obfuscation, or at least of carefully contrived statistics.

Reps are a determined lot. Some offices won't see them. We had to limit it to three in the morning and three in the afternoon. The jostling crowd of reps around the office door as it was unlocked first thing in the morning, each intent on being one of those three, was reminiscent of Walmart on Black Friday.

In the good old days, they brought us tchotchkes like pens, note pads, coffee mugs, calculators, reflex hammers, or my personal favorite, a rubber nose advertising the expectorant Mucinex that blew a green snotty goop out the nostril when you squeezed it. Or, better still, they invited us on all-expenses-paid trips to conferences that just happened to be at a beach resort, golf club, or ski center.

Until 2008. Then, in what is cynically described by Harriet Washington in her book *Deadly Monopolies* as a "very public act of contrition," it all came to an end. Prompted by some physicians and ethicists expressing "concern about the 'relationship of reciprocity' that even a pizza or cheap mug can establish between doctors and drug makers," thirty-eight companies found religion and agreed to clean up their act.

Now they can only supply food and beverages. My Bosnian nurse, Rasima, who runs on coffee, and I would feign interest in the latest product and swear fidelity to entice them to bring us a Starbucks travel pack (not that awful wishy-washy Dunkin' Donuts stuff). Ironically, the reps promoting diabetes medicines usually brought pastries and doughnuts.

Alternatively, these folks clamored to take us to "drug lunches," which I hasten to point out were *about* drugs, not mid-day substance abuse-fueled debauches. Sometimes, they offered a $600 honorarium if you gave a "talk" to your office colleagues regurgitating sales information the rep had fed you earlier.

There were the more elaborate "drug dinners," too. Doctors get wined and dined at some moderately fancy local restaurant with an expert talking about some subject relevant to the company's latest product. Though you occasionally hear things like Reuters.com's report on a drug dinner for three doctors at New York's Japanese restaurant Nobu that ran up a tab of nearly $10,000.

It always seemed to me this was not a very good teaching/indoctrination format. After beating your brains out over eleven hours on rounds and in the office or being on call, it only takes one glass of wine and something to eat to slide in to an amnesic oblivion where it's easy to ignore the "expert" droning on in the background.

Sometimes there are lighter moments, as with the Novartis drug dinner promoting Zelnorm as a miracle treatment for irritable bowel syndrome (that has since been withdrawn from the market). We were shown glossy pamphlets illustrating the Bristol Stool Scale. "Sausage with cracks" through "no solid pieces."

But we're doctors. We don't get grossed out. We took it all in stride and ate heartily while our flagrantly gay, irreverent physician assistant cracked jokes about "pictures of your children."

DRUG COMPANIES KNOW WHAT THEY'RE DOING

Of course, I'm all cold objectivity and not for sale, so all this information the reps and "experts" fed me, along with the over-rich food and wine, doesn't affect my prescribing.

Or that's what I, along with all the other doctors, think. But these perks "foster familiarity and comfort" and a "gift relationship and gratitude," says E. Haavi Morreim, professor of human values and ethics at University of Tennessee College of Medicine.

Talking to the Markkula Ethics Center, she cited a study of ten physicians attending a conference whose prescriptions went up two to threefold for the products presented. She also sites a letter in *JAMA* in which a patient came to the hospital with an infected insect bite. The intern prescribed "a nice inexpensive penicillin." But the resident overruled the intern and favored a more "modern" choice for this "severely" ill patient, deciding he needed a brand new antibiotic at $183 a day.

The supervising attending physician looked into the incident. It turned out the resident had just been wined and dined by a drug rep for the company that made the new antibiotic.

A combined study of twenty-nine other studies corroborated this. When doctors met with pharmaceutical reps (and 94 percent of doctors admit to having some relationship with pharmaceutical companies), rates for prescribing that company's products went up. It's to the point where there's supposedly a $10.60 return for every $1 invested by the company.

Another tactic of the drug companies I've always found a little sneaky is "profiling." This is when pharmaceutical companies get information from local pharmacies "that allows them to track an individual doctor's prescriptions down to the last pill," explains Elizabeth Cohen.

It lets them see if a doctor is playing the *quid pro quo* game and if their wining and dining and tchotchkes are working.

I readily confess I am as much a sucker to these siren drug reps, these quasi-cheerleaders, as my fellow doctors. But I am rather amused, and perhaps perturbed, by a statistic in the July

2005 *Family Practice*, that the more pharmaceutical reps a doctor sees, the poorer his prescribing habits.

COERCING THE PUBLIC

Drug companies realize that while the doctor, in his role as prescriber, is the gate keeper, he's not the actual consumer.

You may have this naive idea that medicines are prescribed for a specific illness when there is a need. But you'd be wrong. Medicines are just another product for which advertisers can increase demand and create a larger market for.

Drug ads are common in magazines. It intrigues me that there are two-page ads for the newest blood thinnner, Eliquis (apixaban), in my copy of *Family Handiman*, and of course for Cialis, with macho handimen and dreamily contented-looking women.

As anyone with a TV is only too aware, advertising medicines is allowed on television in the U.S. It became possible when those clever Congresspeople relaxed the FDA advertising guidelines in 1997.

The U.S. is only one of two countries in the world that allows direct-to-consumer advertising of prescription medicines. The second is not necessarily what you think of as a bastion of aggressive free enterprise. Tucked away in the southern reaches of the Pacific, where "every day is like a Sunday afternoon," it's New Zealand.

Drug companies have found if a patient comes in wanting a particular drug they saw advertised, most physicians prescribe it, even if they feel "it may not be the most effective therapy," notes Bremner.

Shockingly, a harried doctor writes whatever prescription the patient wants 54 percent of the time. I know from experience that giving the patient what he wants is often the quickest, least acrimonious way to get a demanding person out of the office and out of my hair. It can come back to haunt the doctor, though, setting up the expectation in the patient to get whatever he wants like some spoiled child. Doctoring and parenting have a lot in common.

The FDA is meant to review drug ads to ensure they're appropriate. But, as Marcia Angell reports, there are thirty reviewers for 34,000 ads (offering $2 to $3 returns for every $1 spent on TV).

The rest of the world presumably feels like the Brits, who aren't having any of it. The British government points out, rather primly, that the aim of advertising is not to provide balanced information, but to persuade the customer to want a particular product.

EXTENDING PROFITABILITY BY EXTENDING PATENTS

Another maneuver to help sales is for the company to find some way to extend the patent on a drug. In 1994, Congress increased the length of a drug patent from seventeen to twenty years, but companies still find ways to extend exclusivity even further.

One way is suing a generic manufacturer for patent infringment up to five times to get thirty months' worth of extensions. Filing for multiple patents staggered over months or even years, changing to OTC status, doing further testing of the drug on children, and finding a new indication are other strategies used by drug companies.

When the patent on Prozac was running out, Eli Lilly scored an extra three years of exclusivity with the invention of Serafem, "which is simply Prozac used for premenstrual tension," Angell notes. The company also extended the patent by coming up with a long-acting, weekly Prozac instead of the usual daily dose.

As noted, many "new" drugs aren't much more effective than the old. That's because the company hasn't devised anything new, it's just performed some chemical sleight-of-hand, making a minor adjustment to the molecule and marketing it as a new product with a new twenty-year patent.

AstraZenica, manufacturer of the stomach acid-reducing "purple pill" Prilosec (omeprazole)—at the time the top-selling medicine with annual sales of $6 billion—surely had some heartburn about its patent expiring in 2003.

But the clever chemists went to work and found that the mirror image of omeprazole—esomeprazole—also reduced acid (though there's a lot of debate about whether it's more effective). The new drug was marketed with great fanfare as "the new purple pill" Nexium with its own patent.

It was a similar story with Schering-Plough's most widely prescribed allergy medicine, Claritin (annual sales of $2.7

billion). This came off patent in 2002 and went OTC as well. But at about the same time, Merck came out with prescription-only Clarinex, which is claimed to specifically target outdoor allergies after showing no superiority over Claritin for treating indoor allergies.

"All these allergy claims are pretty hocus-pocus," says pharmacologist Raymond Woosley, dean of the University of Arizona College of Medicine, as reported in *USA Today* in 2002. "Indoor allergy vs. outdoor allergy? Come on."

Furthermore, Claritin's generic ingredient (desloratadine) is converted by your body into loratadine, the generic in Clarinex. So "anyone who has taken Claritin has taken Clarinex," says Woosley.

Bill Tauzen, president of the pharmaceutical lobbying organization PhaRMA, seems to epitomize the pharmaceutical industry's delusions of grandeur in overlooking how much of the industry is comprised of "me too" drugs. In an interview in *The New York Times* in 2005, he said, "We don't make ice cream or handbags or automobiles, we make products that save lives."

It would be innaccurate and churlish to deny this completely, but it smacks of industry hubris. Once again, the key is to be informed. Know these fandangles go on and don't think that new necessarily means superior; usually, it just means more expensive.

As a side note, even when a name-brand medicine's patent expires, it doesn't mean the generic equivalent is cheap as dirt. For the first year, one generic manufacturer gets exclusive rights. This company then practices "shadow pricing," keeping the price high simply because it can. It's after that first year the price really comes down.

COOKING UP NEW DISEASES

There are accusations that to expand the market further, the pharmaceutical industry emphasizes or even contrives illnesses to increase sales.

In his book *Manufacturing Depression*, psychotherapist Gary Greenberg suggests that what is really just unhappiness and re-actions to adversity is being turned into depression and a "bio-chemical imbalance" for the sake of selling antidepressant drugs.

The concept of unhappiness as a disease was vigorously pro-moted when the SSRI medicines hit the market. After Prozac was released in 1987, Merck sent out 50,000 copies of a booklet called *Recognizing the Depressed Patient* to "educate" doctors. The PR team excelled in creativity when they came up with a record they called *Symposium in Blue*, with songs like "I Been Treated Wrong" and "I'm on My Last Go-Round," with a drug package insert slipped discreetly into the dust jacket.

Osteoporosis and osteopenia have been heavily promot-ed to sell bisphosphanate drugs like Fosamax, though experts claim the testing we do (with DEXA scans, a lucrative growth industry of its own, both in medical practices and "scan-in-a-van" businesses) doesn't identify women getting bone disease that will cause significant fractures. In other words, the women being identified don't generally benefit from the pharmaceutical course of treatment they then receive.

There are plenty of diseases with which normal symptoms have been "pathologized" and emphasized when some product came on the market to treat them.

Testosterone deficiency syndrome, or male menopause, is one huge growth industry with prescriptions growing nearly three-fold between 2001 and 2011, to nearly $2.3 billion in 2012. In the July-August 2014 *AARP Bulletin*, Steven Woloshin, M.D., a professor of medicine at Dartmouth's Institue for Health Policy and Clinical Practice, calls this "the mother of all disease mongering," with normal symptoms of aging being touted as "low T."

Restless leg syndrome, if not made up, has certainly been greatly promoted by a lot of TV ads since Requip hit the market.

Heartburn (going by the grander-sounding name GERD, or gastro-esophegeal reflux disease) provides a huge market and is played up; women made irritable by their periods are claimed to need treatment for PMDD, or premenstrual dysphoric disorder, which allowed the above-mentioned extension of the patent for Prozac; rambunctious children are diagnosed with ADD or ADHD and prescribed a whole bunch of stimulant variants of amphetamine.

I mentioned coming up with extra off-label uses for drugs as a way of expanding the market. The antiepileptic medicine Neurontin was originally indicated as an add-on for controlling seizures, but shortly before the patent was due to expire, and with the help of small, poorly designed studies and ghostwritten articles, Park-Davis promoted its use for migraines, pain, anxiety, and as a sole medicine for seizures.

THE DOCTOR AS PATSY

This all may give you pause, the ways in which doctors are sold and drugs are treated as nothing more than a commodity. It does me. Pause, if not outrage, especially at what a patsy I've been. Undoubtedly that's part of why I have gone into it in some depth.

You may worry your doctor is prescribing not what's best for you, but what drug companies have persuaded him to prescribe, even if he's unaware of it because it's presented in some supposedly impartial medical journal.

Fortunately, sources exist for your doctor to turn to for unbiased information (excepting that even these sources report on clinical trials that may have been manipulated to advantage). Have a discussion to determine whether he uses these, and if not, encourage him to do so.

One is the drab, monochrome, dull-as-ditchwater but scholarly *Medical Letter*. It contains no ads, no hype, just the facts, conveniently condensed. There's also the Cochrane Collaboration and Medline, both mentioned in *Getting the Right Information*.

An interesting, relatively recent innovation is "academic detailing." It involves an "un-sales force" of reps, many of whom used to be "real" drug reps who have come over from the dark side, who visit doctors' offices with objective, evidence-based information on the best, most cost-effective ways of treating different illnesses. Often this entails generic medicines.

The organization No Free Lunch is trying to counteract the drug industry's influence. It gets doctors to sign a pledge not to see drug reps, and even has its own tchotchkes, or at least No Free Lunch pens they send in exchange for drug company pens.

The government is trying to inject some cold hard truth and objectivity into this whole business of selecting the right treatment. The Affordable Care Act formed the Patient-Centered Outcomes and Research Institute to look at the "relative health outcomes, clinical effectiveness, and appropriateness" of different treatments. The problem is that the $1.1 billion allocated is paltry compared to the $7 billion per year the pharmaceutical industry spends on marketing to doctors.

PROFITS PAST THE ZENITH

I'll temper my criticism of the pharmaceutical industry and their obscene profiteering by saying they appear to have passed their zenith. Their profitability seems to have peaked around 2008. Part of this is the dearth of new products, but mainly it's the phenomenal rise in R&D spending. This is due to a massive increase in the regulations of phase 3 of drug trials, the bit when new medicines are tried out on people. The industry spent $802 billion to develop 139 drugs between 1997 and 2011, and now spends "a staggering $5.8 billion per drug," reports Mathew Herper in *Forbes*.

Genomics—a topic I go into further in *Getting the Right Future*—will likely affect this, making clinical trials more personalized, in a sense. Pharmaceutical companies will probably eventually only be trying out drugs on people they know will react to them. That will make trials much smaller and cheaper.

ADVERSE EFFECTS AND OTHER ADVERSITY

Medicine is a double-edged sword. Those powerful chemicals can do you good, but they can be pretty poisonous as well. This applies to over-the-counter medicines and even natural herbs and supplements (as discussed in the section on complementary and alternative medicine below).

Every year, two million people suffer from adverse drug reactions (ADRs) and 100,000 die, according to the FDA. They are so prevalent that, on average, any hospitalized patient suffers an ADR every day, reports the *Washington* Post, adding that the extra cost for ADRs in just hospitalized patients is estimated at $3.5 billion per year.

In addition to the direct toxic effects, one medicine can interact with, potentiate, or inhibit the effects of others. Some foods do the same, especially grapefruit juice, which can inhibit absorption, and that ubiquitous item so many people self-medicate with, alcohol, which has many dangerous interactions, including potentiating sedating effects.

I remember attendings at medical school claiming you couldn't safely be on more than three medicines because it was impossible to keep up with all the possible interactions. And today, all those little old ladies seem to be on seventeen or more of them.

Bodily factors like age, illness, dehydration, and others affect the metabolism and effectivness of medicines. Environmental factors, like heat and cold, can also have effects.

Sometimes, as with an allergic reaction to a new drug, adverse effects are unnavoidable and catch you by surprise. But the embarassing claim made by "investigative journalist and exasperated husband" Stephen Fried, author of *The Bitter Pill: Inside the Hazardous World of Legal Drugs*, is that the most common cause of problems is the doctor's lack of knowledge regarding drug therapy.

He wrote his book after his wife became "Floxed." That is, she developed delirium, confusion, tremulousness, and visual and cognitive changes lasting weeks and necessitating MRI scans, EEGs, spinal taps, and yet more medicine from a single dose of the antibiotic Floxin. Johnson and Johnson discontinued it as of June 2009, though generic ofloxasin is still available,

"Faulty prescribing often takes the form of failure to observe safety warnings and contraindications," notes Robert W. Donnell, M.D., participating in a roundtable discussion on Medscape. For example, one study showed 27 percent of patients prescribed metformin for diabetes had an "absolute contraindication."

More exactly, 27.2 percent of inappropriate prescriptions are wrong dosage and 24.9 percent are an "inappropriate drug for the condition," reports The Physician Insurer Association of

America (an organization with some skin in the game when it comes to medical errors).

The story of gastric motility medicine cisapride (marketed as Propulsid, another highly profitable medicine) is a good illustration of a certain deficinecy of doctors when it comes to paying heed to warnings. I relate this partly to show I am not the only doctor to ever overlook a "black box" warning.

After cisapride had been on the market for a while, concerns arose regarding electrical conduction problems in the heart, prompting the FDA to send out warning letters. The medical profession blithely forged ahead, prescribing cisapride despite this precaution.

So, the FDA moved to the most severe "black box" warning, so called because of its heavy black border when it appears on a drug insert. It's not to give it a funeral look, presumably, but to catch the doctor's attention. Still, "adverse prescribing persisted despite regulatory action" and the "Dear Doctor" letters, notes Donnell.

A *The New York Times* article of June 2005 accuses Johnson and Johnson of suppressing results of studies showing adverse effects, especially in children (the article says 20 percent of babies in neonatal ICUs were taking cisapride for gastroesophegeal reflux despite no studies establishing its safety in children). The company is also reported to have resisted the FDA's attempts to add cautions to the label and reduce promotion.

Johnson and Johnson finished up agreeing to pay up to $90 million to settle lawsuits eventually involving claims that

300 people died and as many as 16,000 were harmed by taking Propulsid. The drug was subsequently withdrawn from the market, immediately before a public meeting was scheduled for an outside panel of experts to review the evidence.

While you might now expect this sort of behavior from a drug company, it doesn't reflect well on doctors' diligence at heeding warnings.

It's my observation that many people are not particularly aware of the adverse effects medicines can have. But doctors certainly should be. Again, though, it's one of those TMI situations. Yes, there is that pious commandment of the Hippocratic Oath of *primum non nocere* ("first do no harm"), but keeping up with all the harms that medicines can do is difficult.

Hippocrates was smart enough to realize it looks far worse for the doctor if his patient dies because of a prescribed treatment than if his patient dies due to a more passive role taken while managing an "incurable disease."

Take a good look at the long list of adverse effects the pharmacist provides when you fill your next prescription. Pay closer attention to the litany of adverse effects run through at breakneck pace in the course of TV drug ads, which I'm sure the manufacturers hate having to include.

The difficulty of keeping up with ADRs and interactions and warnings was brought home for me when I had to give a deposition about a patient wanting to sue the manufacturer of

Chantix, which he took to stop smoking and claimed it caused neuro-psychiatric problems.

It was a joke. This guy had been my patient for years, and his neuro-psychiatric status was a disaster long before the Chantix. He was the most noncompliant, recalcitrant, alcoholic, pot-smoking, curmudgeonly old bastards you are ever likely to meet. He looked like the Unabomber, with his wild hair and unkempt beard, and he apparently even took a swing at the judge at one of his many court appearances.

In the course of the deposition, I was forced to deny any knowledge of receiving a letter about the new black box warning Pfizer issued when after-market surveillance noted certain neuro-psychiatric side effects of Chantix. With great gusto, the patient's attorney waved under my nose a copy of a receipt for the Dear Doctor letter with my signature on it.

My excuse for not remembering was simply that we get Dear Doctor letters every day, which is just one example of the problem of "overwarning," which the *Archives of Internal Medicine* defines as an "exhaustive list of every reported adverse event, no matter how infrequent or minor."

Management of this kind of problem is ideally suited to a computer, with its infallible memory, immunity from fatigue or distraction, and ability to be ever vigilant, unlike my poor befuddled brain.

But alerts on computerized health records, like anything designed by computer nerds, is taken a little too far. My experience with EHRs is that they take the cake when it comes to over-warning. They sound their alarms so much, and about such obscure ADRs, it's ridiculous.

KNOWING YOUR MEDICINE

Another classic way to get into trouble with medicines is to not know what they are.

It's not uncommon for people to go to appointments with a plastic bag or container with a colorful array of pills and capsules. They're totally confused about what's what. Others ask for a refill saying, "Oh, you know, doctor, the little round white ones." As Kussin points out, there are 3,000 round white pills on the market.

Ideally, you know the brand and generic names of your medicine. I've seen patients taking Coumadin and warfarin, not realizing they're the same blood thinner, putting them in grave danger of bleeding out. Know how much to take and when, all of which is on the original container dispensed by the pharmacist. Bring all your medicines in their original containers to every doctor visit.

Also, some medicines have dangerously similar names. This can be more of an issue for the pharmacist trying to figure out if the doctor's scrawl says Celexa or Celebrex.

It's also common for patients to take medicines incorrectly. Perhaps the most typical screw up is "double dipping" when they forget they already took a dose.

Bad things don't just happen when doctors write prescriptions. There's also the sin of omission, when doctors fail to prescribe something they should.

Experts and lots of compelling evidence urge the use of beta-blockers and angiotensin-converting enzyme inhibitors as the mainstay of heart failure treatment. But they are used "at inordinately low rates," says Donnell. High cholesterol tends to be under-diagnosed and under-treated. Diabetes is often poorly controlled. Cardiovascular disease in psychiatric patients is notoriously under-treated.

BUYER BEWARE

Just being aware (and perhaps a little understanding) of your doctor's difficulty keeping up with everything about every medicine is a good start for getting the right treatment.

Asking whether there could be adverse effects or interactions might avoid problems if your doctor's being inattentive. It just might shift his attention off tomorrow's golf game long enough to realize he's prescribing you something he shouldn't.

It's a buyer-beware situation, requiring you to know about what you're prescribed. When you get home, look up tpossible ADRs and interactions and read the printout the pharmacist gives you.

It's not feasible to provide a comprehensive list of all adverse effects and interactions here, but there are plenty of websites that do. Try UpToDate.com and Drugs.com or the FDA (at www.fda.gov/Drugs/ResourcesForYou/Consumers/ucm196029. htm under the drugs tab). Or, you could go to the more traditional source, the *Physicians' Desk Reference*.

Protect yourself against the similar name issue by knowing the generic and brand name. That way, you know something's up if the pharmacist gave you celecoxib (generic for Celebrex) instead of citalopram (generic for Celexa).

Your pharmacist may well be better informed than your doctor about medicines and their adverse effects and interactions. In fact, it's not uncommon for a pharmacist to save a doctor's ass by picking up on some oversight before the patient comes to grief. You're usually asked when you pick up your medicines if you have any questions, so make use of a good resource and ask about adverse effects and interactions. Make those helpful pharmacy people feel needed.

Avoiding the sin of omission and being sure the doctor's prescribing the appropriate medicines are harder tasks. It requires you know what the best treatments are. As noted in *Getting the Right Diagnosis*, so much is done by rote, by habit, by "that's how it's always been done."

Search online for the name of your condition and *treatment algorithm*. For high blood pressure, for example, the NIH website has the Joint National Committe's algorithm for treatment, which takes you through the recommendations from lifestyle modifications to a list of suggested drug catagories. The Indian Health Service has good algorithms for treating different types of diabetes, including a downloadable PDF (touted as being in "accessible text," so there's a rare bonus).

It should be noted, though, that some experts criticize so called "cookbook medicine" with algorithms.

QUESTIONS TO ASK ABOUT YOUR PRESCRIPTIONS

When you are being prescribed a medicine, ask:

- For the brand and generic names
- What it's for
- For dosage details and when and how to take it (the so-called "sig," an abbreviation for *signa*, meaning "write on label")
- About possible adverse effects and interactions with any medicines, supplements, or foods
- When it will start to show results and what you should expect
- How long to take it and if refills are available
- Whether anything needs to be monitored, like having a pro time blood test with Coumadin/warfarin or a blood count with methotrexate
- What to do if you miss a dose

GENERICS ARE JUST AS GOOD

A quick note about generic medicines is in order, as they are often an important part of the "right" treatment, particularly given how much more affordable they are. This also means your insurance carrier may be insistent on a switch to a cheaper alternative.

A lot of people doubt that generics are as good as name brand medicines. This is not the case, though.

"Brand-name drug manufacturers have gone to extraordinary lengths to mislead doctors, pharmacists, and the public into believing that their products are produced to higher standards, and thus are safer and more effective than the same drugs produced by generic companies," charges the watchdog organization Public Citizen on its Worst Drugs/Best Drugs website.

The FDA has no doubt that generics are good. Not only are they 80 to 85 percent cheaper, the FDA website tells us, they are required to have the same active ingredient, strength, and bioequivalence (they must get into the blood stream and be as active at the receptor site), and they must be shown to perform the same. "Research shows generics work just as well as brand name drugs," the FDA reassures.

TAKING YOUR MEDS LIKE GOOD BOYS AND GIRLS

Former U.S. Surgeon General C. Everett Koop profoundy observed that "Drugs don't work in patients who don't take them."

Getting the right medicine is essential, but it won't do you much good if you don't take it and take it in the right dose, at the right times, and avoid potential interacting substances.

Noncompliant patients make their doctors a little crazy, but they're a fact of life in the trade. "Only about 50 percent of patients actually follow their prescription plan," notes Topol.

It's a serious problem. Up to 11 percent of hospital admissions, 40 percent of nursing home admissions, and about 125,000

deaths annually are due to noncompliance, according to the American Pharmacists Association.

It's not just the noncompliant patient who can be hurt. Failure to take pills as intended, with treatments for TB and HIV for example, contributes to development of drug-resistant bugs. Exposing microorganisms to nonlethal doses of antimicrobial medicines, like by taking them too intermittently or stopping them too soon, breeds resistant "superbugs" like methicillin-resistant *Staphylococcus aureus* (MRSA) and multidrug-resistant tuberculosis (MDR-TB).

Being on a regimen involving medicines multiple times daily for the rest of your life is difficult. I can barely remember to take an antibiotic twice a day for ten days. And, dare I say it, people in hostels or jails or the kind of places where you see more TB aren't always the most conscientious patients.

Some people don't take their medicines because they can't afford them; the WHO says one in five prescriptions aren't filled because the recipient can't pay for it. Some patients don't think they really need them. Others are worried about adverse effects or just plain forget.

There are low-tech solutions for forgetting, like the popular weekly pill organizers, which also help stop people from over-dosing because they forgot they already took their pills. These do mean removing medicine from its original container, though. Keep at least one pill in its bottle for identification.

More sophisticated technologies can help, too, like the talking pill bottle holder made by MaxiAids (www.maxiaids.com).

A doctor, pharmacist, patient, or family member makes a voice recording of instructions on how to take the medicine. MediVox Rx Technologies makes a medication reminder, and "Glow Caps" go on your medicine bottle and flash and make noise when it's time for your medicine. They also order refills automatically and can send updates to family or friends.

Many devices tattle on you if you ignore them, sending an e-mail to your doctor. Some insurance companies and pharmacies also contact the doctor's office if a patient fails to refill a medicine.

If half my patients are not properly compliant with their regimen, that could be an awful lot of notifications, and a whole lot more parenting.

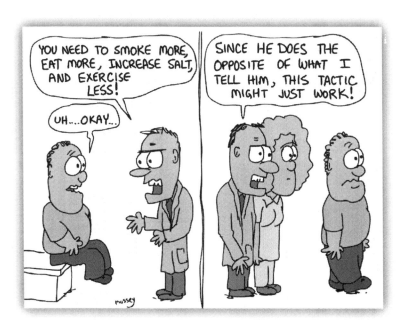

TREATMENT WITHOUT MEDICINE

Medicines are the most common form of treatment, but there are many other nonpharmacological forms. They often seem more wholesome and natural, enhancing your own body's powers of healing (though they're often used in conjunction with drugs).

For a quick look at some of the major categories, there's:

- Physical therapy (PT) treats musculoskeletal problems like sprains and strains and arthritic, siezed-up, or damged joints (particularly in the neck and back). PT is also often used after orthopedic surgery to regain function. For more detailed information, go to "For the public" at the American Physical Therapy Association's website at www.apta.org.
- Occupational therapy (OT) is a hodgepodge of treatments and gadgetry to help people be as functional and independent as possible. It helps with a range of physical, neurological, and mental problems to restore or preserve activities necessary to daily living. OT can be very helpful in advising how to modify the environment or developing particular skills in the elderly and people with disabilities to keep them leading as normal a life as possible. Visit the American Occupational Therapy Association at www.aota.org.
- Speech therapy helps people with use of nerves and parts of the throat and respiratory system that control speech, and helps treat brain dysfunctions in people with speech defects, like stuttering or following a stroke. Speech therapists are also often called on to assess difficulties with swallowing (people in danger of aspiration

pneumonia) and are often consulted by neurologists and pulmonologists, and they may be part of a PT/OT program. Learn more at the American Speech-Language-Hearing Association site at www.asha.org.

- Cardiopulmonary rehabilitation is for people with a heart or lung disease like coronary artery disease and is especially important after a heart attack and to build up exercise capacity and cardiovascular strength with heart failure. It will usually be prescribed by a cardiologist. See the National Heart, Lung and Blood Institute website at www.nhlbi.nih.gov.

- Respiratory therapy (RT) deals with breathing and lung issues. Practitioners treat all age groups, including young kids with pulmonary problems, like Cystic Fibrosis and asthma, as well as the elderly and people with chronic lung diseases like COPD (emphysema). Oxygen therapy, breathing treatments, and postural drainage are standard tools of the trade. Therapists oversee ventilator use in hospitals, and some work in patients' homes. Most of the websites I found are about becoming a respiratory therapist. For general information, Wikipedia has a good page at en.wikipedia.org/wiki/Respiratory_therapy.

- Nutritional therapy/counseling is offered by many people, lots of whom lack training or qualifications, but instead have a bug up their asses about some wacko diet. Registered dietician nutritionists (RDNs) have an undergraduate degree in nutrition and postgraduate training and pass a qualifying exam overseen by the Academy of Nutrition and Dietetics. Nutritionists are becoming sub-specialized, with focuses like cardiac dietitian, nutritional support dietitian, sports nutritionist, diabetes educator, and kids or old folks. They advise on nutrition for general health, weight loss and gain, and augment other treatments for problems like diabetes, high cholesterol, obesity, gout, kidney stones, and osteoporosis. The best overview I found is called the Better Health Channel at http://www.betterhealth.vic.gov.au. Follow the path Healthy living > Food and nutrition > More about food and nutrition > Dietitians.

- Psychotherapy helps you sort out emotional issues. Talk therapists are usually psychologists or licensed clinical social workers, though your spouse/friends/family/dog (no joke; animal-assisted therapy is all the rage these days) can provide informal "psychotherapy" by listening and being loving and supportive. Psychotherapy has lots of variants and techniques for stuff like anxieties, phobias, PTSD, and coping with difficult life situations. A lot of people find this preferable to taking psychotropic drugs, though you may be crazy enough to need both. There's a lot of good information at the website of Psychology Today at www.psychologytoday.com.

Then there's surgery, of course, which is the next most common treatment after drugs. Finding the right surgeon is much the same as for any other doctor, so follow the advice in *Finding the Right Doctor.*

Check your surgeon's basic credentials (see the American College of Surgeons at www.facs.org) and ask about previous experience. You probably don't want to be the first person the surgeon has ever done this operation on. Check into results, too; a surgeon should have statistics on how many of any given operation he's performed and occurrence rates of complications.

Before lying down under the knife, ask a few questions. Do you really need the operation? What happens if you don't have it? What are the alternatives? What's the post-operative care going to involve? How much pain and disability is there likely to be, and for how long?

COMPLIMENTARY AND ALTERNATIVE MEDICINE

WHAT IS IT?

So you've been plugging away with your doctor, taking those expensive, poisonous, manufactured chemicals. You've been sliced and diced by some knife-happy, madcap butcher. But you're not better.

This situation, and many others, can prompt an interest in CAM (as mentioned in the *Introduction*, there's a newly emerging trend to say complementary and integrative health).

Allopathic "Western" medicine is what regular doctors practice, at least in the West. It slavishly adheres to the dogma of evidence-based medicine. It's what we doctors are taught in medical school, though this is changing some despite the pharmaceutical industry's push to keep everything focused on manufactured medicines.

CAM is a diverse group of medical and healthcare systems, practices, and products not generally included as part of conventional allopathic medicine, according to the website of the National Center for Complementary and Integrative Health (NCCIH). It's basically anything that's not in the conventional Western doctor's bag.

The borad field embraces a lot of different modalities. Many are relatively well-known, like acupuncture, acupressure, naturopathy, osteopathy, chiropractic, meditation, herbalism, homeopathy, shiatsu, aromatherapy, and biofeedback. Then there are weird things like gua sha, bioresonance therapy, reiki, auriculotherapy, moxibustion, craniosacral therapy, crystal healing, and the Feldenkrais Method.

Overall, CAM has four main categories:

- Biologically based therapies use natural ingredients to promote healing, as with homeopathy, herbal remedies, supplements, and specialized diets
- Energy-based therapies manipulate your body's energy fields with needles, light, sound, electromagnetic, or other interventions, like acupuncture and its variants
- Manipulative or movement-based therapies include practices such as osteopathic, chiropractic, massage, tai chi, and yoga
- Mind-body therapies employ mental manipulations to affect physical health, as with meditation, guided imagery, and biofeedback

Many CAM practices use a combination of techniques. Native American healers use herbs and belief systems, while yoga and tai chi have physical and meditative components, for example.

There is a tendency to talk about CAM as a single unified entity. But it's a whole spectrum, and trying to talk about or judge it as one thing is as meaningless as talking about "illness" as one disease. In assessing safety and efficacy, consider the pros and cons of each different modality.

Despite the fact that few CAM treatments are backed up by clinical evidence for their efficacy, CAM is popular. A study back in 1993 reported in *NEJM* estimated more people went to CAM providers (425 million) than primary care physicians (338 million) in 1990. A 2002 National Health Interview Survey found 62 percent of U.S. adults used some form of CAM in the past year, and it's reported to be a $28 billion per year industry.

Many people use some kind of CAM in a minor way without necessariy thinking of it as such. They've applied aloe to a burn, taken melatonin to get to sleep or St. John's Wort for stress, used glucosamine supplements for joint pain, or supplemented with ginseng for energy or ginger for dyspepsia.

CAM is more likely to be used by women and the highly educated. Often, those who turn to it have chronic, inflammatory, arthritic, or allergic conditions, or conditions with vague, hard-to-understand probems for which allopathic medicine doesn't have much to offer (and are often thought to have a significant psychological or somatization component). The latter would include things like fibromyalgia, fatigue, non-specific joint pains, lupus, irritable bowel sydrome, back pain, Lyme disease, and chronic headaches, to name a few.

A lot of CAM therapies strike many of us as a little alien and weird. However, many "normal" or mainstream treatments of today started out as "natural" alternative therapies. Aspirin from willow bark, digoxin from foxgloves, atropine from belladonna, and poppiess that produce opium—and thus morphine, codeine, etc.—are some examples.

For a good overview of this strange new world, I recommend the National Institute of Health's wonderful NCCIH website at nccih.nih.gov. It covers the whole subject from soup to nuts, all in a far more comprehensive way than I can here.

MET WITH CONDEMNATION

A lot of potential CAM patients wonder what their doctor's reaction will be if they broach the subject.

When I came to the U.S. and was doing a residency in New York, I did a rotation at a travel medicine clinic at Cornell. One day, the doctor there was particularly confrontational with patients. I was a greenhorn straight off the boat and didn't realize this was just part of the charm and normal interaction of New York. But this guy was full of himself and condescending. That is, he was being a doctor.

He was examining one patient who asked him, "What do you think of this iridology business, doc?" Obviously not knowing about it, he asked the patient, "What is that?"

The patient explained, "You look in the eye at the iris, as a window to your bodily health, and can tell what's wrong with the different organs by variations in the color and form of the iris."

Without a moment's hesitation, the doctor's response was "A crock of shit."

Now, I find the concept of iridology a little wacky and wouldn't put much store in it without some convincing literature. But I was impressed by how this doctor, totally ignorant of the subject, had absolutely no reservations expressing instant and unqualified condemnation.

Unfortunately, this isn't such an unusual response from allopathic doctors. Probably in large part because of this, many patients keep it a secret that they're using some form of CAM. In fact, *NEJM* reports 70 percent of patients using CAM therapies don't tell their doctors.

This isn't good.

Full Disclosure To Your Doc

It isn't good because your doctor needs to know.

If it is truly to be complementary, it requires working as a team with your doctor. If he's some bigot who thinks anything that doesn't come promoted by a drug rep is hocus-pocus, understandably you might be inhibited about telling him. But there are compelling reasons to clue him in.

Ma huang (also known as Ephedra) is a wonderful Chinese herbal tea that will put lead in your pencil. But the ephedrine it contains can give you seizures, high blood pressure, irregular heartbeat, or even a heart attack if your ticker's already a little dodgy. Ginkgo biloba can play hell with blood thinners, as can ginseng, glucosamine, and a bunch of other supplements, and it may interfere with oral contraceptives, creating a significant complication nine months down the road.

The many possible interactions with conventional medicines necessitate your doctor know what you're taking and getting into. Either talk him around—the NCCIH website has a specific section on talking to your doctor—or move on to a more sympathetic cove.

Things are changing, though, and medical schools are be-ginning to incorporate CAM training. This was largely spurred by a 2002 White House Commission on Complementary and Alternative Medicine Policy report recommending across-the-board integration of CAM into government health agencies and the nation's medical education, research, and insurance systems.

Still, the mindset and education continues to heavily focus on the allopathic culture. This is of course aggressively pro-moted by players like the drug companies, which have a huge financial interest.

SAFETY AND EFFICACY ISSUES
Safety is a concern with any remedy, no matter how "natural." Even physical treatments like manipulation can be harmful (neck manipulations have been known to damage arteries in the neck on rare occasions, for example). So it's just as important to inform yourself about safety and efficacy issues as with al-lopathic treatments.

CAM is a less regulated, lesser-known entity. A lot of people are troubled by the question of "How can one begin to sort out the quack stuff?" as one little old lady put it to me.

Some call all CAM therapies "quack stuff." Many allopaths point to a lack of adequate scientific evidence, and some claim too much testing has used flawed methodologies.

A few of the better established therapies, like acupuncture and chiropractic, have been subject to proper clinical trials, however. Acupuncture has received a tentative endorsement by the NIH, and the WHO reports it can be useful for abdominal pain, adverse effects of chemotherapy, alcohol detox, allergies and other purposes.

Critics often claim the benefits are not meaningful, or that treatmetns merely provide placebo effects. Though this prompts the somewhat philosophical question of whether it really matters if it's a "real" or "fake" improvement, if it eases suffering. But more on this and the pacebo effect below.

The National Library of Medicine reports on forty systemic reviews of a variety of CAM treatments including acupuncture, massage, naturopathy, and yoga between 2002 and 2007. It found that of these, only 25 percent offered "sufficient evidence to conclude that a given CAM therapy was effective for a given condition."

The NCCIH notes "Rigorous, well-designed clinical trials for many CAM therapies are often lacking; therefore, the safety and effectiveness of many CAM therapies are uncertain." But

"NCCIH is sponsoring research designed to fill this knowledge gap by building a scientific evidence base about CAM."

A detailed look at a lot of evidence is found in the book *Trick or Treatment* by science journalist Simon Singh and Edzard Ernst, M.D., Ph.D., "the world's first professor of alternative medicine." This well-informed book does seem to have a negative take and condemns virtually all modalities.

The Cochrane Library and the Cochrane Reviews (www.cochrane.org/cochrane-reviews) are a reliable place to review clinical trials and findings related to CAM treatments. The Cochrane Collaboration Complementary Medicine Reviews is a useful resource.

The section on "Resources for Healthcare Providers" at www.medlineplus.gov takes you to a lot of studies listed under different topics. There's also a section of PubMed with NCCIH-funded studies, though some get a little arcane (trying out herbs on arthritic rodents, for example, in a study whose title honors that great gobbledygook tradition: "Celastrus treatment modulates antigen-induced gene expression in lymphoid cells of arthritic rats").

The objection that CAM is all snake oil because it's not proven by clinical trials is just the oppressive dogma of the pundits of "evidence-based medicine," claim CAM supporters. They say CAM invokes a completely different science, it's a different system of medicine, with forces at work that Westerners don't understand.

Standardization of methods is necessary for clinical trials, and CAM proponents point out that this isn't reasonable because treatment isn't just from one ingredient or component; it's a culmination of the whole package, including not just the remedy, herb, or modality used, but also the interaction with the therapist, lifestyle alterations, diet, environment, and so on.

Clinical trials also require comparison with a placebo, which presents some hurdles in the realm of certain CAM treatments. For example, how do you have a placebo for various types of manipulation?

Plus, clinical trials cost a boatload. Without the deep pockets of a pharmaceutical company and the promise of a highly profitable, patentable product, no one's going to spend millions on testing.

Supporters also say the longevity of CAM proves its merit. Many CAM treatments have been around for mellinia. The Greeks and Romans used spinal massage. Otzi, the 5,300-year-old Bronze Age "Ice Man" found frozen in a glacier on the Austro-Italian border, had herbal medicines in his possession. He had some interesting tattoos too, on acupuncture points, prompting speculation they are therapeutic markings. This suggests acupuncture is much older than the 3,000 years previously thought.

The "belief in holistic principals and the notion of nurturing of vital energy as the way to health" just makes intuitive sense, says a report by a group of Australian naturopaths. "I don't need a 2-million-person, double-blind, randomized trial to tell someone to eat blueberries because they are low in sugar and high in antioxidants," says Dr. Mimi Guarneri, medical director of Scripps Center for Integrative Medicine.

We don't have a great handle on efficacy. But what about safety?

On the whole, CAM treatments are less likely to cause adverse effects than allopathic drugs, but many people have the mistaken belief that because something is "natural," it's automatically safe. That's not so. Plenty of poisonous stuff grows naturally; just ask any mycologist.

Hopefully, your CAM practitioner knows what's what, but it's smart to look up adverse effects for yourself. NCCIH's site has a limited list of adverse effects of some natural treatments at https://nccih.nih.gov/health/herbsataglance.htm. Wikipedia also has a list at en.wikipedia.org/wiki/List_of_herbs_with_ known_adverse_effects, or just search for the name of the substance you're interested in. Keep in mind all that stuff about finding reputable sites covered in *Getting the Right Information*.

To reiterate, an important part of reducing risk is to let your doctor know exactly what you're taking and/or doing.

Another big concern is about the purity and standardization of remedies and supplements. My local paper just ran a report of FDA inspections that found violations in half of the manufacturing facilities, with such charming extras as rodent urine and rat turds in the supplements. They also found a liquid multivitamin supplement containing 40,800 micrograms instead of 200 mcg of selenium per dose, which caused everyone's hair to fall out.

Supplements and remedies, though under the jurisdiction of the FDA, are not regulated as medicines. They are regulated as foodstuffs and not subject to the same strict standards of efficacy and purity as prescription and OTC medicines.

Reduce the risk by buying products blessed by the United States Pharmacopeial Convention, which bear the USP seal on the packaging. This body verifies supplement identity, quality, purity, and strength. It does not mean a product will be effective; it doesn't guarentee it will do what you or your CAM practitioner want, just that it is what it says it is and it's pure.

CHOOSING A PRACTITIONER

Choosing the right CAM practitioner may be more crucial than choosing your allopathic doctor, as the "therapeutic relationship" is often a more significant part of treatment. Much of the information in *Getting The Right Doctor* applies, but here's some CAM-specific advice.

If your doctor is sympathetic to CAM, he may be able to make a recommendation. However, his ability to advise you is dependent on how informed he is. And unfortunately, a lot of allopaths—myself included—never learned much about complementary and alternative stuff.

Most doctors know zilch about CAM from medical school. So, unless yours has an interest in it or is willing to learn about it (in an already overwhelmingly busy life, which I think I've complained about already), don't expect a whole lot. Again, things are changing, but it's too little too late for me and many others.

The CAM practitioner himself should be able to advise you whether his modality is right for you. Hopefully, you've found one ethical enough to say, "Sorry, this isn't the right treatment." But, like the surgeon with his predilection for surgery, a therapist may be enamored with his own particular form of treatment and think it good for everyone.

There is some safeguard in some states requiring certain alternative therapists to be licensed, which involves training courses and exams, and so imparts some credibility. Professional organizations of CAM therapists provide information on standards of practice and training, and state licensing requirements for the different states. They can help locate practitioners, as well.

These sites, like the practitioners, may be just a tad enthusiastic and uncritical about their particular art. For example, the banner across the top of the page on one homeopathy site proclaims, "Of course it works!"

These organizations can be located by doing a search under the specific therapy. A few helpful addresses include the Federation of Chiropractors Licensing Board at www.fclb. org, the National Certification Commission for Acupuncture and Oriental Medicine at www.nccaom.org, the American Association of Naturopathic Physicians at www.naturopathic. org, and the Directory of Health Organizations at dirline. nlm.nih.gov. The NCCIH site also has a detailed section on finding a practitioner and credentialing information for different states.

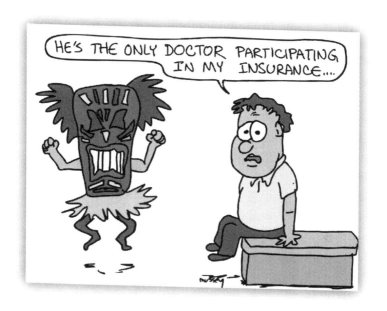

ADDITIONAL INFORMATION

A word on exactly how to look things up online might be helpful.

You can approach your research by starting with what you want fixed and looking to see what CAM treatments have been tried for that. "What will help my irritable bowel?" Or you can approach it from the specific treatment. This may be less helpful for finding out what to do about a particular illness but is more applicable for prevention. "Should I take a vitamin E supplement?" or "Would omega-3 fish oils help me?"

Probably the best way to search is to inquire whether a particular modality helps a specific problem. "Will tai chi help my arthritis?" or "Will reflexology treat my kidney failure?"

Of course, there are countless junk sites out there with worthless information about CAM. *Getting the Right Information* can help you sort out the reputable from the rest. In particular, be wary of sites that sell anything.

The WHO has a list of questions for deciding if CAM is right for you. Some might be hard for you to answer and might more appropriately be put to your doctor (assuming he's not being a bum about it and is cooperating). They are:

- Is the therapy suitable for your condition?
- Does the therapy have the potential to prevent, alleviate, and/or cure symptoms or in other ways contribute to improving your health and well-being?
- Is the therapy or herbal medicine provided by a qualified traditional medicine/complementary and alternative medicine practitioner or health care practitioner with adequate training, background, skills, and knowledge, preferably registered and certified?
- Are the herbal medicinal products or materials of assured quality and what are the contraindications and precautions of the products or materials?
- Are the therapies or herbal medicinal products available at a competitive price?

Last Word

CAM has the disadvantage of not having as much science-based evidence behind it as allopathic medicine, and people are also put off because they can't understand how it works. There's no anatomical basis for the meridians postulated by acupuncturists; calculation shows there's not a single molecule of the original substance still present in the more dilute remedies of homeopathy; there is no anatomical or physiological reason for why chiropractic treatments enhance circulation as claimed.

On the other hand, CAM practitioners usually have a much more holistic approach with better appreciation for the mind-body connection. They investigate the whole person, lifestyle, and circumstances. They tend to spend much more time with their patients, too, and are generally better listeners who project a lot more caring.

CAM is usually more of a partnership, with the patient far more involed in treatment decisions. Many people also appreciate that they can buy herbs, remedies, and devices for themselves without prescriptions. So CAM definitely fits in with the idea of emancipated, informed, self-sufficient patients who take charge of their healthcare.

Even if it's all just belief in the ritual and "liturgy" of needles, manipulations, exercises, herbs, potions, and mystique, I say if it seems to work and it's not doing you any harm (which includes not bankrupting you), then it doesn't matter what the mechanism is. If you feel better, who cares why?

THE PLACEBO EFFECT

As you probably know, a placebo effect is the benefit people experience from a treatment simply because they believe it's going to do them good.

The placebo effect can be the sole reason something works. The nay-sayers claim this is the case with most CAM treatments.

It can be useful and enhance the effectiveness of any therapy. It's typically greater when there's ritual or a mumbo-jumbo factor, which is where CAM practitioners sometimes win out over allopaths, with their accupuncture needles, burning cones of moxa, massage with hot oils, manipulations, and exotic herbal preparations. This is likely to have a much greater placebo effect than just swallowing a pill.

The phenomenon also causes drug manufacturers all kinds of grief. When they have to do drug trials comparing with a placebo (which many people say is a woefully inadequate standard—but that's another story), the placebo is often quite effective.

In his book, Greenberg notes that in a total of seventy-four trials on twelve leading antidepressants, only thirty-eight showed an advantage over a placebo. Another analysis showed the drugs improved the HAM-D score (the psychiatric symptom scale that indicates severity) by ten points, but the placebo did so by eight points. That means the placebo "is 80 percent as effective as the medicines," Greenberg points out.

When Effexor first came out, the rep (this time one of those square-jawed, hail-fellow-well-met guys) brought the standard glossy brochure with all the stats and pictures of a woman sitting alone, staring wistfully over a sunlit pond (why she's not home doing the wash or preparing dinner, I don't know).

But if you look carefully, the stats showed minimal difference from the placebo. "Placebo's pretty damn effective," I pointed out, at which the rep rolled his eyes.

The placebo effect has been recognized by the medical profession for years, but has been treated as an embarrassing quirk it's best not to talk about. The idea of intentionally giving patients placebos was ruled unethical, though giving someone an expensive pill with the potential for dangerous side effects that is no better than a placebo seems to me the more ethically questionable option.

There's also a reverse placebo, or "nacebo" effect, which is when you experience an adverse effect because you believe it to be a likely result of doing or taking something. The nacebo effect seems to be the basis of reportedly successful voodoo and witch doctor hexes. But, there is also the danger your pharmacist is hexing you with that long list of all the awful things your medicine might do to you.

I remember prescribing Xanax for a patient's anxiety, but the list of possible side effects made her too anxious to take it.

Many things play into your belief that you'll get better, and thus the placebo effect, as well. One significant factor is seeing someone you have confidence in. Another is being treated with something you believe in, which is more likely if you're involved in the treatment decisions.

TREATMENT EXPECTATIONS

Any doctor can have biases, misinformation, misconceptions, brain farts, bad days, and other obstacles to providing you with perfect treatment. It's not a bad idea to try to decide for yourself what you need. Ultimately, a treament plan should be formed in collaboration with your healthcare provider.

Despite my vignette about doctors prescribing whatever curries favor with the raunchy drug reps, the usual reality is that doctors carefully weigh the pros and cons of any treatment, though they may do it almost subliminally.

As mentioned, it seems quite a lot of people aren't attuned to the concept of adverse effects. I was once like that about aspirin, which was used for every possible ailment in our family when I was a kid, and we had no thought of it doing anything bad. I recall being flabbergasted at medical school when a physiology professor told us he had a friend who died of a gastrointestinal bleed caused by aspirin.

All treatments have potential down sides. Even non-pharmacological and CAM treatments can have adverse effects, even if they're just the expense or inconvenience. Any treatment or test requires a risk-benefit calculation (just like tests, as discussed in *Getting the Right Diagnosis*).

One thing that can help, bringing in a little objectivity, is when there's some kind of grading scale or algorithm to evaluate the ratio between possible risks and benefits.

I was just away at the Southern Unitarian Universalist Summer Institute (a sort of camp for grownups with some spiritual stuff thrown in for those who want it). A good friend, who was also a counselor/guide, fell down a small waterfall on a hike. He was admitted to the hospital, primarily because he was found to be in atrial fibrillation (an abnormal heart rhythm with potential to form blood clots that can float off and cause a stroke or other problems). Does he need to be on blood thinners for the rest of his life (which is not a benign treatment because it can cause dangerous bleeds in your GI tract, brain, and other places)? Decisions like these cannot be made capriciously.

In this instance, the CHAD scoring system looks at the factors relevent to the patient's risk. It considers things like whether you have congestive heart failure or hypertension, whether you're over 75 years old, whether you have diabetes, and whether you've had prior strokes or mini-strokes. It provides a score, and if a patient gets less than 2, he only needs a simple medicine like aspirin instead of a full-fledged anticoagulant.

Most cancers have some kind of staging dependent on the type and how much it's grown or spread. Then there are usually five-year survival stats with different kinds of treatments for any given stage to help make rational decisions.

Ask your doctor if there is such a scoring scale for what ails you or for any of your treatment options. A lot of conditions don't have a scale, which sometimes leaves things in a subjective realm. The number of variables, like your age, overall health, how active you are, cost, availability, the seriousness of your condition, what may happen if you don't treat, and others all muddy the waters.

As mentioned, ask about adverse effects and in what ways you'll need to be monitored with a particular treatment. If you're having surgery, ask about potential complications and their likelihood, as well as what's to be expected during recovery. Ask about the shortcomings any treatment may have.

And remember, you can get sucked into a treatment that might not be best for you if the doctor stands to make extra money from it.

It's also important to have a clear idea of what to expect from your treatment, particularly to create realistic expectations and help you recognize when it isn't working. In my experience, plenty of patients have unrealistic expectations, especially about how long treatment will take. They often expect results much quicker than is reasonable. Patients aren't patient.

People expect to be cured the next day with antibiotics, but these medicines typically take about 48 hours to start working. Everyone wants their antidepressant to make them happy within days, but they usually have to be taken for four to six weeks before having any effect. Talk to your doctor about how long it should take to see results. If, after that time, things aren't improving, discuss the possibility that your treatment isn't the right one.

Another unrealistic expectation is that everything can be cured. With many diseases, the best you can do is manage the symptoms.

Your back pain may not ever go away completely, but it can be alleviated, allowing for a better quality of life. Like numerous conditions, Parkinson's disease can be slowed down a bit, but not cured.

Expecting to be cured of an incurable disease can cause a lot of strife.

The doctor makes risk-versus-benefit calculations, and just through force of habit and because most patients take a pretty passive line, he'll make a decision. Yes, you should have your arthritic knee replaced rather than taking arthritis medicine. No, your acne isn't bad enough to warrant the risks of taking Accutane. Yes, it's worth the extra cost to get a twice-daily dose of amoxicillin instead of the three-times-per-day dose available at Walmart for $4. Yes, it's worth the potential damage to your liver to take Lamisil to clear up your toenail fungus.

That's how it goes, unless you jump in and show your interest.

CHAPTER 5

GETTING THE RIGHT PRICE

———————

SO MANY STORIES, AGAIN

THE COST OF HEALTHCARE IS a crisis. It's a major contributing factor in about 60 percent of individual bankruptcies, despite 75 percent of these people having health insurance, according to Trisha Torrey in *You Bet Your Life!: The 10 Mistakes Every Patient Makes*. But it's also bankrupting corporations, retirement funds, and the nation as a whole as it nears 20 percent of our GDP and eats more and more of our collective lunch.

Healthcare often causes insurmountable hardship for those who get ground under the wheels.

Consider Alice, a loving wife whose husband Steven was dying of lung cancer. She couldn't deny his wishes as he "kept saying he wanted every last minute he could get." But those precious minutes landed her with medical bills totaling $902,452 (with a United Healthcare insurance policy that maxed out at $50,000).

Or...

A patient getting a nerve stimulator implanted for back pain at Mercy Hospital in Oklahoma City didn't ask the price. He was scheduled for surgery as a day case in a hospital that was part of the Catholic Sisters of Mercy, whose pious mission is "to carry out the healing ministry of Jesus." He had $45,181 left in his insurance policy and figured, "how much could a day at Mercy cost?" He got his answer: $86,951. That included $49,237 just for the nerve stimulator, on which the hospital charged a 150 percent markup. He ended up paying over $40,000 out of pocket.

Or...

When Amanda Bennett's husband was dying of kidney cancer, his doctors thought he just needed comfort care, yet he still ran up bills totaling $91,115. Of that, $14,022 accrued in the last three days of life, as Bennett relates in her book *The Cost of Hope: A Memoir.*

Or...

A patient with non-Hodgkin lymphoma was told the cancer drug Retuxan was the only thing that would save his life. He paid $13,702 *for a single dose*, though it only cost the administering hospital about $4,000 to buy and the manufacturer probably around $300 to produce.

These stories are all too common in American medicine. Most of the above were told by Steven Brill in his emotive article, "Bitter Pill: Why Medical Bills Are Killing Us" in the March 2013 edition of *TIME*. In it, he minutely dissects various medical bills and "follows the money." I shamelessly borrow these examples because he was right on the money, if you'll allow the pun, perfectly illustrating what the industry has become as patients receive enormous bills while healthcare vendors make massive profits.

Numerous factors contribute to this fiscal millstone. The good news is, once you gain some insight into them, opportunities to reduce your healthcare bills come to light.

MY QUALIFICTIONS AND EUPHEMISMS

I consider myself doubly qualified to advise you on reducing your personal healthcare costs. I'm a doctor and therefore have firsthand experience with how these bills come about. But I'm also a practiced cheapskate, as my kids will readily attest, though I've always tried to impress on them that "parsimonious" is the preferred term.

As a cheapsk—parsimonious individual—I feel your pain, spending your hard-earned money on boring stuff like medical bills when you could be buying some necessity like an Aston Martin Rapide S or a getaway beach house. Even those cost a lot less than the medical bills some people end up with.

WHAT'S WITH THESE PRICES?

Brill wonders why a trip to the ER for what turns out to be indigestion costs more than a semester at college and why the blood tests done during a few days in the hospital cost as much as a car. You've probably stared dumbly in awe at a medical bill or two yourself. Why is it like this?

As Gerard Anderson, a healthcare economist at the Johns Hopkins Bloomberg School of Public Health, puts it, "All the prices are too damn high." Don't these high-flown academicians ever tire of their overly technical, incomprehensible explanations?

But there's more to it than just those damn prices.

ASSIGNING BLAME FOR RUNAWAY COSTS

Patients blame the doctors and the hospitals. They do too much—whether it's to make more money, to justify their existence, or because they're afraid of missing something and getting sued—and then they charge too much for it all.

Doctors blame the patients. They always want the latest and greatest of everything, they want ever more tests and treatments, and they have unrealistic expectations.

Everybody blames the system, with its "healthcare by the yard" fee structure. And, of course, there's the legislative fandangling that tilts the field in favor of the vendors, making healthcare so profitable it's more an investment opportunity for corporations than a healing art practiced by parties concerned with quality of life and social justice.

CONSUMER CONTROL OVER SPENDING

You might expect a dissertation on staying healthy and preventive care to keep your healthcare costs down. It works, but that's not what I'm talking about now. I'm focusing on exercising some control over how much you consume and how much you pay for it by being an informed and involved patient.

There are limits to what you can do about the asking price of any health product or service. But you do have influence in many instances, and you have even greater say over what you buy in the first place. Introduce some moderation to a system that, for various reasons, tends to do too much.

Compounding excessive consumption of expensive healthcare products has been the fact that many Americans are uninsured. This is changing with the Affordable Care Act (ACA), a mandate for coverage and a step toward bringing the U.S. more in line with the rest of the industrialized world—and not a few developing nations—with nationalized or universal healthcare systems. It's something the World Health Organization calls "a widely shared political aim of most countries."

Despite the ACA, there will still be significant numbers of uninsured and underinsured. They'll still be paying out of pocket, as will many others who have insurance but haven't met their deductibles, who have a large co-insurance, who have some condition that isn't covered, or who otherwise get stuck with some or all of a bill.

Doctors always seem to assume you have some Cadillac insurance plan that covers everything. They blithely order tests and write prescriptions without a thought for the cost. If you're a self-pay patient, make sure your healthcare providers know it.

OUT-OF-POCKET HEALTHCARE EXPENSES

Healthcare coverage may now be obligatory, but it isn't simple. The decisions you make regarding your coverage plan can greatly affect your premiums and out-of-pocket expenses.

A disclaimer: I'm not an insurance expert, and health insurance is becoming an ever more complicated business. There are plenty of experts around, though they often want to sell you a policy. But to help see where you might reduce expenses, I offer a brief outline and explanations of some of the jargon; so much involved in insurance and medical billing is a triumph of obfuscation.

With conventional insurance, you go to any provider (a doctor, nurse practitioner, physician assistant, hospital, radiology department, lab, physical therapist, rehab clinic—whoever you get some kind of medical care from), and the insurance company picks up the tab.

Except they don't pick up the whole tab. Insurance companies negotiate a discounted payment, knocking off a certain percentage of the total bill. This is an arcane business, with each insurance company negotiating its own secret fee scale with each provider.

Then, there are other costs you assume on top of your premium. Your premium, as you probably know, is what you (or your employer) pay each month for continuing coverage. There's your deductible, the amount you have to pay before your insurance kicks in. Deductibles typically start at a few hundred dollars, but a lot of newer plans are hitting up to $5,000 to $6,000. The higher your deductible, the lower your premium.

You may have a co-payment, a generally modest amount you have to pay for each doctor visit or other encounter. It's usually around $20, and you're meant to pay it at your visit. This a source of some strife in doctors' offices, when patients claim they don't have money, a check book, or a credit card and want to be billed. Paying someone to generate and send that bill can cost a doctor $20 or more. A common gripe in the doctor's lunchroom is that nobody expects to go to the supermarket without money. This is why the bulletproof glass your doctor's gracious but unbending receptionist sits behind is festooned with charming signs telling you "Your co-payment is expected at the time of service."

There's also coinsurance, a percentage of the bill you must pay, even after meeting your deductible. This is usually 10 to 20 percent of the cost. So, if your insurance approves a $60 payment for some service your doctor provides and you have a 10 percent coinsurance fee, you pay $6 and the insurance pays $54. It may not sound like much, but if you have a major inpatient procedure and 20 percent coinsurance, things can get pretty hairy.

Note the "if your insurance approves a $60 payment" above. An approved amount is how much the insurance company thinks a particular service or product is worth. It may be a whole lot less than what the doctor is asking. If you go to an "in-network" provider, he's already agreed to accept this discounted amount as a sort of *quid pro quo* for getting the insurance company's business. But if you go to an "out-of-plan" provider, you may have to pay the difference between the asking price and the approved amount.

A safeguard against being bankrupted by coinsurance is the limit on out-of-pocket expenses. After you shell out this amount, your insurance pays 100 percent of approved amounts. But check the fine print; this may not apply to all aspects of coverage.

The ACA has abolished two features of health insurance that seriously worked against consumers in the past. One was the lifetime cap, or the maximum amount your insurance policy would ever have to pay out. The other was the preexisting condition exclusion that provided insurance companies with practically endless loopholes to deny coverage or payments. Now, you can't be denied healthcare coverage because you were reckless enough to develop some problem like diabetes or cancer.

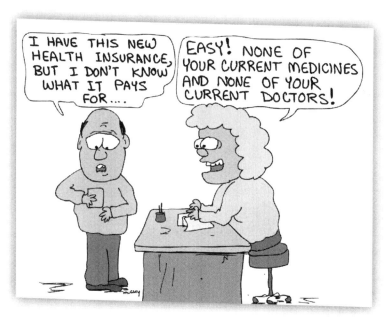

WADING THROUGH COVERAGE OPTIONS

To pick an appropriate plan, you need to decide which type best meets your needs. There are a lot of them out there, but here's a quick look at the major types.

There's the traditional "indemnity" style, otherwise called fee-for-service (FFS). Some wags claim it stands for "fend for yourself." Doctors get paid for each service they provide. Of course, this encourages them to provide lots of services. This type of plan gives you the most freedom as to what healthcare providers you go to. The billing process is the most complicated and deductibles, co-pays, and coinsurance have profound effects on your premium.

Managed care is a cheaper but more restrictive form of coverage. You're bound to an in-network primary care doctor for services, products, and referrals. Your insurance carrier also usually has to pre-approve expensive tests and treatments. That makes for some ruffled feathers when some bean-counter at the insurance company tells your doctor no.

Health maintenance organizations (HMOs) are a popular form of managed care. You have an exclusive primary care physician whom you have to go to for everything. He must give you a referral if you want to see a specialist. This is the most restrictive arrangement, but consequently usually has the lowest premiums. Because doctors are paid by capitation—a set amount for a particular patient over a specific time frame—their incentives become quite different than with FFS structuring.

The next most restrictive form of managed care is the preferred provider organization (PPO). You can go to an in-network provider who's paid on an FFS basis, or you can go to an out-of-network provider, but you'll be on the hook for more out-of-pocket costs.

One hybrid of HMOs and PPOs is called a point of service plan (POS). That might not be what you normally use these initials for—but it may hint at the kind of coverage you end up with if you're not careful. With a POS, you can usually go to whomever you want, but you pay more for out-of-plan providers. There's also an exclusive provider organization (EPO), where you have to go to the company's in-network providers.

Variations on how you pay your premiums can help keep costs down. Health savings accounts (HSAs) and flexible savings accounts (FSAs) let you pay out-of-pocket medical expenses with pre-tax dollars (it's taken out of your pay by your employer, reducing your taxable income). Deciding if this would be advantageous for you depends on many things, particularly how much you pay in taxes; seek individualized advice. These kinds of plans are sometimes referred to as consumer-directed healthcare (CDHC) because you have more involvement in deciding how much of your savings account you're willing to spend. It's all in keeping with the new age of the in-charge, self-directed patient.

Of course, there's Medicare for old people—those over 65, if the acrimonious wrangling over Federal expenditure doesn't result in the threatened raise in the age of eligibility. Some doctors and medical groups have formed accountable care organizations (ACOs) with the innovative method of paying the providers by a form of capitation based on patient outcomes and cost of care. The idea is to provide incentives for good, cheap care.

Medicaid is the other government-run insurance program. It's mainly for the poor, but it also covers some kids, pregnant women, elderly, and disabled people. To qualify, you must have an income around 100 percent of the federal poverty level (FPL)—an annual household income of $24,250 for a family of four in 2015.

The ACA sought to expand eligibility to those earning 133 percent of the FPL. But it's all become politicized and states with governors and legislatures that don't like the ACA haven't increased Medicaid eligibility. This created a class of people too poor to qualify for ACA subsidies toward insurance premiums (if you earn below 133 percent of the FPL, you aren't eligible for subsidy, as it's assumed you have Medicaid) but who earn too much to qualify for Medicaid in their states.

The working poor often really get the shaft. They make up a lot of the patients at the Moss Free Clinic. The ACA has created five insurance plan tiers: bronze, silver, gold, platinum, and catastrophic. People who can only afford the most basic bronze plan may still have significant out-of-pocket expenses. This can easily lead to hardship and even bankruptcy.

Some people can afford health insurance but opt not to buy it. They gamble on not getting sick or hurt, or at least not *too* sick or *too* hurt. The prediction is that lots of people will choose to pay the relatively small penalty the ACA imposes for not taking out insurance.

Insurance is a gamble. I did a rough calculation of how much I paid out in health insurance premiums during the 24 years I was with the medical group I recently retired from. I came up with $157,000. I compared that to how much the insurance shelled out, which looks to have come in under $10,000. It seems I would've done much better to have kept my money. Like "the house," the insurance companies always seem to win. That's not to say they can't spare you a major financial crisis, though.

If you think it a stretch to consider insurance a form of gambling, you won't make it with Allah. Muslims consider it a form of usury, which is forbidden. This has prompted some conflict with the mandated insurance of the ACA. However, a Muslim has a duty to see that people have access to healthcare, so several prominent Islamic organizations support the act.

Carriers also feed on our anxieties and risk aversion, selling us insurance against more and more tenuous risks. Tom Jones insured his chest hair, Dolly Parton her boobs, others have insured against alien abduction, and three sisters in Scotland paid $150 a year to insure against immaculate conception.

You can hedge your bets with "catastrophic insurance," partly self-insuring with a large deductible—say $5,000—to greatly reduce your premium. If you do this, you're liable for all that money before the coverage kicks in, but it can save you from going completely broke if something goes really wrong.

CHOOSING AN INSURANCE PLAN

Choosing a plan is a highly individualized process. Considerations like how much you're willing to pay out of pocket, how much of a gambler you are, and your risk factors for getting sick—which include things like your medical history, family history, environment, and lifestyle choices—all matter.

With implementation of the ACA came the healthcare exchange, the marketplace where you compare different plans. Head to your state's site if it has its own exchange or to the seamlessly launched national site www.healthcare.gov, which has a lot of information about health insurance in general and about picking a plan. Any health insurance agent should be able to give you the run down, too.

Most importantly, pay attention to whether a plan lets you see the providers you want to see. But also find out whether there are restrictions on coverage of extenders (nurse practitioners or physician assistants), whether it will cover you overseas if you travel, and exactly what peripheral services (like physical therapy and chiropractic) it covers.

The National Committee for Quality Assurance (www. ncqa.org) provides a report on health insurance companies; go to "Directories," then to "Health Plans," and then to "Health Insurance Plan Rankings" for an assessment of about 1,400 insurance plans. Also, review the opinions of other consumers about particular health insurance plans through the National Association of Insurance Commissioners and Consumer Reports. The Patient Advocate Foundation (www.patientadvocate.org) also has a lot of information to help you choose an appropriate plan and to help with many aspects of your health-care in general.

As a side note, maybe you feel bad for the insurance companies, shackled with all these new ACA regulations. After all, they now have to take on the added potential expenses of anyone and everyone, even if they have pre-existing conditions; they can't set lifetime limits on what they pay out anymore; and they can't just dump anyone who becomes too expensive anymore (as has been their charming habit before the ACA). Take some comfort from the Pricewaterhouse Coopers findings published in the July 2011 Health Research Institute Report concluding that the ACA—which the insurance companies have so vigorously opposed and complained will force large premium hikes—will boost their revenue by up to $200 billion by 2019.

EXPLAINING THE EXPLANATION OF BENEFITS

If you're one of those happy souls with insurance (which is supposed to be all of you, now that the ACA is in effect), your provider sends a bill for the [often excessive] fees. As I'll get to soon, these charges are often fantasies. But the insurance company pays a markedly discounted amount—the approved charge. Approved charges are a murky business, with insurance companies negotiating individual contracts with different providers; all parties tend to be secretive about this stuff. Regardless, the approved amount is invariably significantly less than what's billed.

The provider may also send you the whole bill at this stage, but usually the first item you receive is a statement showing the total bill, what your carrier paid, and what your portion is, or an "explanation of benefits" (EOB).

This is one of the industry's droll jokes. "Explanation" is such a flagrant misnomer for this horror-show of obfuscation and mass of cryptic abbreviations, codes, jargon, and multiplicity of terms for the same thing. It is not unusual to find your EOB completely incomprehensible.

A nuclear stress test, for example, is listed as "NM MYO REST/SPEC EJCT MOT MUL." Or, after a recent visit to an orthopedic hand surgeon, I received a classic EOB; all it said was, "99214 est pt detailed" and "73140 fingers."

Knowing something about medical billing, I worked out that "99214" was the code for the office visit (although a level-4 visit with a charge of $185 for the cursory exam of my finger seemed a little over the top, but that's just standard "upcoding," which I'll get to soon). The "73140 fingers" was the procedure code for the X-ray of my finger.

It's a bit of a stretch to call this an "explanation" of anything. I suspect if it was in the interest of the participants to have everyone understand their EOB, somehow it could be done. I think we would all be even more outraged at charges if it weren't for the obfuscation, though.

INSURANCE CODE-SPEAK

Every medical bill has two vital components: a diagnosis, indicated by an international classification of disease (ICD) code, and a procedure, indicated by a current procedural terminology (CPT) code. "Procedure" might conjure something dramatic like a heart transplant or brain surgery, but an office visit, with all the history taking and fondling that goes on, any test, or just about any other thing done to you is considered a procedure.

There's also the healthcare common procedure coding system (HCPCS), which is the same idea as the CPT code, but specific to Medicare. It covers a broader range, including things like ambulance rides and surgical supplies. And there's the diagnostic related group (DRG) code, which is like a cross between an ICD and a CPT code for hospital use. It's used in a capitation-like system, with the hospital getting paid a defined amount for each DRG code.

An ICD code contains five digits, providing enough combinations for a specificity verging on the absurd. A slightly wacky pediatrician in the group I was with liked say it was her ambition to diagnose an E845.0. That's a "fall in or from a spacecraft." Not from a plane or a train or a skateboard or a boat or a car. Not from a building or into a manhole or a well. Not from slipping, tripping, or stumbling. These all have their own different codes.

The CPT is also comprised of up to five digits. It tells your carrier what services were provided., which determines that all-important business of how much a doctor should get paid. Again, the five digits allow for an exquisitely detailed description.

For example, the codes 58180, 58200, and 58210 refer to three types of hysterectomies. The differing last three numbers indicate such variations as whether lymph nodes were excised or the fallopian tubes removed. A 58260 is a vaginal hysterectomy, but only if your uterus is under 250 grams. And so it goes, in fastidious detail to describe any and all procedures.

Office visits account for the vast majority of procedures for office-based primary care doctors. Charges vary depending on whether you are a new or established patient and the degree of complexity involved in taking your history, examining you, and making necessary decisions about your care.

Incidentally, to get paid for anything, the doctor has to adequately document what he did. It's a time-consuming pain, but as the legal eagles say, "If it wasn't documented, it wasn't done." Charging for any procedure without proper documentation is considered fraud, even if the doctor really did it.

In our group, if we tried to charge a level of care that the documentation didn't justify, we got a visit from Fran or Terry. It was the job of these two assertive ladies to keep us all out of trouble with Medicare and insurance companies by not allowing submission of potentially fraudulent claims. They would come and lean on you a little, and point out why such-and-such was a level 3, not a level 5... it was a bit like a visit from the Mob.

It's not uncommon for doctors to inflate the complexity of the encounter, adding a little documentation to reflect a level of care beyond what was actually performed. Documentation with a few computer keystrokes has certainly made bill enhancements easier. Not such a boon to those paying the bills.

The coding strikes me as symbolic of medicine's evolution away from the touchy-feely personal business it should be, reducing each patient to a couple of numbers. It's like the old joke, "There's a gall bladder in room 415." Instead of a person, you've become 574.2 (gallstones) needing a 47570 (cholecystectomy).

DENIED!

A great irony of the U.S. healthcare system is that if you don't have insurance—usually because you're too poor to afford it—you get charged more than your neighbor with insurance. That's because you don't have the insurance company fighting in your corner to negotiate a deep discount.

But even the insured sometimes end up with hefty bills. Your deductible and coinsurance may be to blame. Or, your claim may be denied. This sometimes occurs because a particular service or procedure—cosmetic surgery, for a common example—isn't covered by your policy. Remember to call your carrier and study the fine print before an elective procedure or anything you're not sure about.

The most common reason claims are denied, however, is a technical snafu in which some information about you or your insurance was entered incorrectly. Or, if you have more than one insurance carrier, sometimes the wrong one gets billed first.

Your claim may also be rejected because of an incorrect ICD code. If it indicates some diagnosis that's not covered, that may cause the insurance to reject it. To check on whether your bill's ICD code is right, use Find-a-Code at www.findacode.

com/search/search.php. Enter the code or your diagnosis and confirm that the code on your bill matches what's wrong with you.

An alternative is the Center for Medicare and Medicaid Services at www.cms.gov/medicare-coverage-database/staticpages/icd-9-code-lookup.aspx. Here you get the ICD code by putting in a description of the condition, but it requires correct and precise wording. Speak like a doctor; use "pyelonephritis," not "kidney infection," for example. The site can be a little challenging if you don't know the right jargon.

Codes that aren't covered get entered simply because your doctor's busy and distracted, or because he doesn't realize it's not covered. If you contact him about your denied claim and he's co-operative, some creative re-coding may get your claim approved.

For example, sometimes mental health services aren't covered. After all, mental health is the redheaded step-child, always singled out for inferior coverage, though this is another thing the ACA addresses. If your doctor uses 311, the code for nonspecific depression, your claim may get rejected But, if he's creative and uses 309.0 instead—an adjustment disorder with depressed mood—it's probably covered.

There's always an appeals process for denials, though every insurance company handles it differently. Rand Corporation found "Patients who appealed denied insurance claims were successful in getting their cash in more than half the cases, and in more than 90 percent of denials involving emergency care," as

Michael Roizen, M.D. and Mehmet Oz, M.D. report in *YOU: The Smart Patient: An Insider's Handbook for Getting the Best Treatment.* You can request a formal review, or, if you're getting nowhere, contact your state's Department of Insurance and request an independent external review.

People who have been through this emphasize the importance of good records. Don't learn this lesson the hard way. Be paranoid and OCD and assume you are going to have problems. Keep all your medical records and billing information organized from the beginning.

If you're sick as a dog and/or going through some debilitating treatment like chemo, waging war with your carrier is the last thing you feel like doing. If you just don't have the chutzpah, consider a billing advocate.

MEDICAL BILLING FANTASY LAND

No matter why you're responsible for a medical bill, the numbers can be downright terrifying. That's especially true if you don't realize that most charges—especially from a hospital—are insanely inflated, to the point of fantasy. It's vital to understand this, and that you can pay way less than the scary number at the bottom of the page.

In Brill's investigation, he explains that hospitals base charges on what they call the "chargemaster." But he couldn't find anyone to explain what justifies the prices given by the chargemaster. "There seems to be no process, no rationale, behind the core document that is the basis for hundreds of billions of dollars in health care bills," he wrote.

Another point Brill makes is that it's difficult for you to discern what the price should be for different items. There's a conspiracy of silence making it hard for anyone to know what constitutes a reasonable charge. It's often enforced by the contractual arrangements pharmaceutical and medical device companies demand, preventing hospitals from revealing what they pay for a product.

Medicare aims to pay cost plus 6 percent, arguing that not-for-profit hospitals—which most are—shouldn't need a higher markup. Looking at what Medicare pays (more on this further down) gives you a good idea of a reasonable price, though even the government has trouble determining a reasonable base charge.

Some examples of crazy charges Brill cites include:

- $195.50 for a troponin blood test (for suspected heart attacks). Medicare pays $13.94 for it.
- $7,997.54 for a nuclear stress test. Medicare pays $554 for it.
- The patient mentioned at the beginning of this chapter who died of cancer, and whose wife was left with a bill of $902,452, was charged $6,538 for three CT scans that Medicare would have paid a total of about $825 for.
- Even the piddling stuff is grossly overcharged. Examples are $7 each for alcohol wipes when you can buy 200 online for $1.91; and $1.50 per pill for 325 mg acetaminophen

tablets, when you can buy 100 generics for $1.49 on Amazon.

Even the paltry sum Medicare shells out is high by international standards. For example, Medicare pays 71 percent more than the going rate in Germany for a head CT scan, reports Brill.

Despite the mere 6 percent markup from Medicare and the deep discounts taken by private insurance companies, even nonprofit hospitals (80 percent of U.S. hospitals are nonprofit, which means they don't pay taxes) do indeed turn a profit.

Take MD Anderson Hospital, which is part of the University of Texas. It brings in an "astounding" profit margin of 26 percent on revenue of $2.05 billion, according to Brill's *TIME* article.

All that profit is almost a problem, since hospitals don't have shareholders to distribute the money to. They have to be creative. They expand. They buy up competitors and practices (54 percent of physician practices were owned by hospitals in 2012, up 22 percent from ten years earlier). They build (Brill likens the glittering skyline of the 1,300-acre, 280-building Texas Medical Center campus in the distance to Dubai).

They pay their officers huge salaries. Ronald DePinho, president of MD Anderson, had total annual compensation of $1,845,000 and can still "maintain financial ties with three principal pharmaceutical companies," reports the *Houston Chronicle*. The Virtua Marlton Hospital in Philadelphia is part of a four-hospital chain that, in its 2010 federal filing, reported paying its CEO $3,073,000.

My local *Free Lance-Star* reported that the CEO of Mary Washington Hospital, a comparatively small (425-bed) nonprofit, earns a not-too-shabby $600,000 to $900,000 annual salary, along with a healthy bonus of $3 million for his pension fund in 2012. That in spite of his hospital being some $8 million in the hole that year.

The 20 percent of hospitals that operate for profit certainly rake it in, too. Industry giant Hospital Corporation of America (HCA) just built the Spotsylvania Regional Medical Center in Fredericksburg in typical opulent style. Despite HCA being "badly shaken by a wide-ranging Medicare fraud investigation that it eventually settled for more than $1.7 billion," reports *The New York Times*, the 163-hospital corporation not only survived the recent recession, it thrived. It made a 25 percent profit in the last quarter of 2012, according to NewsInvestors.com, benefiting three sponsoring investment firms, including Mitt Romney's infamous Bain Capital.

Further proof of the fantastical insanity of hospital billing is the huge discrepancies in charges from one institution to another, as discussed in the *Introduction*.

FIGHTING THE FORCES THAT DRIVE UP YOUR BILL

Even if you have a solid gold insurance plan, you'll still probably be faced with medical bills. There's always merit in keeping them down as much as possible, but especially if you don't have insurance.

Many places along the healthcare road (superhighway?) present you with choices. You have choices about the quantity of goods and services you consume and choices about whether you go for expensive or cheaper tests and treatments. What you choose can make a staggering difference in the cost.

An informed, assertive patient influences the decisions about their healthcare and is spared many unnecessary expenses. For a better understanding of where and how you can keep your costs down, it's probably easiest to separately address some of the different factors that drive up medical bills.

Factor 1: Innovation

"The dynamics of the medical marketplace seem to be such that the advance of technology has made medical care more expensive, not less," notes Brill. It doesn't mirror most other industries, where prices tend to drop as technologies become more commonplace.

It seems everyone wants the latest, greatest tests and treatments. Of course, the latest aren't always the greatest; not a few innovations have stumbled after a promising start. All those creative boffins in the medical field keep coming up with new stuff, and the more they invent, the more we're inclined to use the stuff, increasing cost further by increasing quantity.

Some of this is driven by patients. Few are content with a good old-fashioned X-ray these days. People with a bum knee, for example, demand an MRI scan—a trend corroborated by a study published in the June 2012 *JAMA* reporting the number of MRIs quadrupled (incidentally, CT scans tripled and PET scans went up 57 percent) between 1996 and 2010.

These tests aren't cheap. New Choice Health (a good place for help finding healthcare prices, at www.newchoice-health.com) tell us a lower extremity MRI—the order to get a picture of the knee—costs $1,500, whereas an X-ray costs $220. The *JAMA* study notes Americans now spend an estimated $100 billion per year on medical imaging.

Expensive, innovative treatments have really taken off with the new "biologicals" developed through elucidation of the genome, but more on that in *Getting the Right Future.* These push the frontiers of treatment, but also the prices. Soliris, a new class of a monoclonal antibody drugs for treating Paroxysmal Nocturnal Hemoglobinurea (PNH, if you prefer), probably takes the cake with an annual price tag of $409,500. Or, as with the case mentioned at the beginning of this chapter, one man with non-Hodgkin Lymphoma paid $13,702 for a single dose of the anticancer drug Rituximab.

Consumers often insist on "nothing but the best," believing they always need the latest innovation. One effective way to keep your bill down is to accept something that isn't necessarily the latest. Do your research. Ask your doctor whether you can get results that are just as good with older, cheaper options.

Newer isn't *always* more expensive, though. Trends like minimally invasive "keyhole" surgery through scopes allow shorter hospital stays or even outpatient surgery, which is much cheaper. The proliferation of urgent care centers provide a cheaper alternative to ERs, though I have reservations about these, as noted in *Getting the Right Doctor*.

Factor 2: Personality And Routine

There are lots of reasons doctors order more than necessary. He may be overly cautious and deathly afraid of missing something, or of getting sued. If he's a consultant, he may feel the need to justify his existence. If he's an ER doctor, he may be stuck thinking this is his one and only shot. Some doctors are eager to please, wanting to send patients out feeling like they've gained something, even in early stages of diagnosis or treatment; similarly, they may be reacting to the impression that patients *expect* to walk out of the office with a prescription in hand.

Other times, your doctor is ignorant of the value—or lack of it—of a test or treatment, ordering it in the spirit of "doing everything," with the hope something might provide some benefit. He may be unaware of the cost of what he's ordering. A study published in *JAMA* in April 2007 found "Physicians do not routinely consider patients' out-of-pocket costs when making decisions regarding expensive medical services." This tends to be compounded by the attitude that "It's all covered by insurance, so what the hell." But this isn't always the case, of course. Plus, when insurance companies have to pay more, that cost is ultimately passed on to patients as increased premiums.

It's not just doctors who inflate healthcare consumption, though. Some patients demand more and more. It's often out of anxiety, which is understandable in many cases. If you push your doctor to do ever more, realize you're also pushing up your bills. Put your emotions aside and have frank conversations with your doctor to keep your expectations and demands realistic.

Much is also mindlessly ordered by doctors as a matter of routine, without careful consideration of the need. This is particularly true in hospitals, where standing orders often exist for daily blood draws, chest X-rays in the ICU, and the like. And the same is true of certain treatments.

My friend Lynne told me of having to refuse the hospital's dose of Dulcolax to help her move her bowels after childbirth. It's routinely given on standing orders. But preferring natural stuff, she just wanted the prune juice her husband was bringing her. Of course, her refusal didn't prevent her from being billed for the Dulcolax, but more on the emotive subject of billing errors below.

Communication deficiency prompts plenty of orders, too. It's often more expedient to do a test again than to get records from another doctor or institution. Prevent this with your own copies of test results.

Remember to tell your doctor if you're uninsured or have a high deductible or coinsurance payment. Explain that you're not expecting a bunch of interventions, and that you prefer as few as possible that offer the most potential benefit for the lowest prices. Ask for explanations of why tests and treatments are being ordered, and if alternatives were considered. If you're in a hospital, ask if you're being given anything on standing orders (a good clue is when the phlebotomist or X-ray technician keeps showing up like clockwork). Inquire about the cost of whatever your doctor is ordering. If you're ever too out of it, appoint a relative or friend to be your advocate and ask these questions for you.

Factor 3: Money On The Side

There are sometimes more devious reasons doctors order more stuff, motivated by profit. Many doctors and medical groups have a financial interest in or own imaging departments, labs, surgical facilities, physical therapy groups, or whatever.

The group I was with owned their own imaging equipment. My fellow doctors and I were pressured to find reasons for patients to get MRI scans, CT scans, nuclear stress tests, and the like, using our own radiology facilities, of course. At the end of the month, it was like a lottery draw for those who had chipped in for a share in these "ancillaries." Sometimes the doctors took a loss, but usually there was a respectable surplus to supplement the earnings they actually worked for.

Lots of orthopedic groups operate a physical therapy department they refer patients to. Dermatologists give Botox injections. Internists run weight-loss clinics and sell nutritional supplements. Neurologists set up sleep labs to diagnose obstructive sleep apnea. Incidentally, OSA seems to be a disease *du jour*, maybe because it requires profitable testing to diagnose.

Rest assured, these coves find compelling reasons why their patients need their particular generally high-priced remedies or services. These extras aren't usually covered by insurance. And there's good evidence that profits are the primary motivation.

For example, in April 2012, the *Wall Street Journal* published a piece about urology groups with their own labs. The piece noted that "Doctors' practices that do their own lab work bill the federal Medicare program for analyzing 72 percent more prostate tissue samples per biopsy while detecting fewer cases of cancer than counterparts who send specimens to outside labs."

To make a tangentially related point, facilities associated with a hospital are usually the most expensive. Independent imaging departments, ERs, surgical centers, labs, etc. are usually cheaper. And, obviously, outpatient is invariably less costly than inpatient whenever feasible.

As discussed in *Getting the Right Treatment*, some doctors get kickbacks from drug or medical device companies for using their products. This is most common with pharmaceuticals, but also prevalent among orthopedic surgeons working with companies making joint prostheses.

Investigate whether your doctor receives any kind of payments from drug companies at projects.propublica.org/doc-dollars. I'm not aware of a similar way to learn about surgeon relationships with medical device manufacturers, though.

It's a bit of a delicate issue, but consider asking your doctor straight out if he receives any incentives to prescribe certain tests or treatments. And though it seems somewhat confrontational, inquire whether he or his group owns or has a financial interest in any secondary provider you're referred to. You might be able to dig up the connection with some online research, too, if you prefer a subtler approach.

Factor 4: Upcoding

Another shifty practice is to "upcode." It's often easy to push the level of service a little to charge more, especially with office visits. Your doctor can make your case out to be a bit more complicated than it is or put down more history or do a slightly more involved exam than is necessary, or even document a more thorough exam than was performed. These justify a higher code with a higher price tag.

I point this out because it's fairly common, but there's not much you can do about it. Only you and your doctor know what went on in the exam room (mind you, all sorts of things go on in the privacy of the exam room that shouldn't, but I defer to your imagination). You probably don't know if your visit was a 99213—worth $107 for my zip code, according to Healthcare Bluebook—or a 99214, worth $163.

Factor 5: The Network

Beware of going to out-of-network providers. You'll be on the hook for much more—or all—of the bill. Plus, the bill will probably be considerably higher than the discounted price the insurance company has negotiated with its in-network providers.

The *New York Daily News* reported in March 2012 about a man who needed brain surgery and went to an in-network hospital. But the surgeon himself turned out to not be a pre-ferred provider and billed the guy $40,091. The insurance company only picked up $8,386, leaving the patient to foot a balance bill of $31,704. You might be forgiven for asking why there was such a huge discrepancy between what the insurance thought the surgery was worth versus what the surgeon thought it was worth.

Just because a hospital is in your network, that's no guarantee everyone working there is too. During a hospital stay, you're usually cared for by a bunch of doctors and consultants you never see or specifically ask for, plus an anesthesiologist, pathologist, radiologist, "old Uncle Tom Cobley and all." That's an Englishism you can Google if you like.

Also, confirm that any services you receive are covered by your insurance. I had a patient, Linda, late 50s, a timid but talented artist and recovering alcoholic who was passed on to me by tennis partner/slightly goofy Lutheran minister/substance abuse councilor/friend Joe. He had shepherded her through the rigors of the intensive outpatient program at the local psychiatric hospital and developed a soft spot for her. Before moving out of state, he entrusted her care to me, for which I was flattered.

Linda had asthma and was recovering from a bout of pneumonia, and her pulmonologist referred her for pulmonary rehab. One of the clerical staff at the rehab unit wrongly informed her that Medicare would cover the service. She wound up stuck with a bill for about $10,000, which she and her disabled husband could ill afford.

She was so timid and uncomfortable haggling with the hospital (the local hospital I referred to above, where the CEO's annual salary was usually the better part of $1 million) that she didn't raise any kind of protest or try negotiating the price down at all. She just paid this king's ransom.

When confirming that certain providers or services are covered, don't take anyone's word for it except your insurance company's. And try to get it in writing.

Factor 6: Billing Errors

As if paying what you're meant to pay weren't enough, it's too common for bills to be inflated by errors.

When I needed an eye exam to get new contacts, I made an appointment with a local ophthalmology group (where I referred a lot of patients over the years, and was thinking they'd welcome me as a VIP). I go in and whip out my Medicare card and the rather brusque receptionist tells me, "Contact lens exams are not covered by Medicare." I don't know why not, but I guess it's like dentists, who somehow sidestepped the whole Medicare thing. "It's $150," came the terse response to my bold pricing inquiry.

When I was done with the technician and playing with the eye charts, the wacky eyeglasses with multiple lenses, and the slit lamp, and after a very brief and cursory visit from the ophthalmologist, the receptionist confronted me with a bill for $250.

Having been forewarned, I questioned this. The receptionist looked irritated and disappeared into the back of the building, then came back and told me in an unapologetic and perfunctory manner, "The doctor hit the wrong key on the computer." If I hadn't been paying out of pocket, I doubt I would've even paid attention.

This was a simple, minor example of a billing error, but one that jacked my bill up by 66 percent. Of course, I later found out I could have gotten the exam for half the price at For Eyes right down the road from this fancy ophthalmology office.

But my story is absolute chicken feed compared to others, like one cited by Brill, in which Scott S. was admitted to Texas Southwestern Medical Center with pneumonia. A thirty-two-day stay landed him with a 161-page bill for $474,064. He owed $402,955, because his insurance had an annual limit of $200,000 and he'd already made claims that year.

As some savvy people with such killer bills do, Scott used a billing consultant who found $113,000 was erroneous and should never have been charged. It included items like $5,890 for saline solution to keep his IV line open and $65,600 for the management of oxygen—both "items that are supposed to be part of the hospital's general room-and-services charge," said the consultant.

"As many as eight out of ten bills for healthcare services contain errors," claims Medical Billing Advocates of America. "If you've ever spent time in a hospital, you've almost certainly been overcharged," says independent hospital bill auditor Edward Waxman of Edward R. Waxman & Associates. "There is no way to avoid being over billed. It is going to happen. In the last several years of looking at hundreds of bills, I've run across only one hospital bill with no errors," he says.

A pretty damning accusation. Carefully scrutinize every bill, especially large ones and especially those from a hospital. Don't be content with a summary, which is usually what a hospital sends, at least at first. When you're sick and feel like crap, you might not be eager to go through your bill with a fine-toothed comb or to get in a fight with your healthcare or insurance provider, but it may pay dividends. Another option is to use a billing consultant, but more on that later.

SAYING NO TO YOUR DOCTOR

If your doctor orders a bunch of expensive tests or treatments but you're dubious about how worthwhile they are, it puts you in an awkward spot. If you speak up, you may come across as questioning his judgment. Or, you might think it unwise to question the professional in the situation.

If you have insurance, your carrier has the same cheapskate instincts as you, but is in a stronger position to demand the doctor justify the interventions by obligating pre-authorization. Of course, this offends the doctor's ego, and "pre-auths" are the subject of much ranting and raving. But they can help dissuade the doctor from a costly step.

Start by asking your doctor to explain the pros and cons of what he's suggesting. It's reasonable to expect a civilized and satisfactory response. If you don't get one, this might not be the guy for you. Be sufficiently informed about whatever you're in disagreement about to politely and rationally question what's being proposed. If you're on the spot, say you want to think about it and go home to read up on the intervention in question.

When declining something your doctor wants to do, provide fact-based reasons for refusing. Suggest alternatives or a compromise, like, "How about an MRI scan if it hasn't got any better in two weeks?"

If your doctor is suggesting alternative treatments, especially through a sideline business, look into the supporting evidence. Many of these treatments lack solid scientific evidence to back them up, so this might be a good out for you in these circumstances.

Saying no is hardest if you have some life-threatening illness and the expensive treatment the doctor recommends may just save your life. Go broke or die; not good options. But if the treatment is not the right one, you may leave your family broke *and* die.

THE GREAT PRICE MYSTERY

Whether you're shopping around because you need some medical procedure or you're fretting over a massive bill you ran up and are wondering if you can get it discounted, knowing the right price helps. But that's easier said than done.

As mentioned, the chargemaster prices are a joke. In her book, Bennett notes a CT scan varies from $776 to $2,586, depending on who paid. A simple appendectomy was $1,500 in one place in California but $183,000 in another, she reports.

The Obama regime recently shook things up, when, for the first time, the Centers for Medicare and Medicaid Services released how much American hospitals charge for the 100 most common inpatient procedures billed to Medicare. The report shows some staggering swings, like admission for chronic obstructive pulmonary disease (COPD) costing $7,044 in one hospital and $99,690 in another less than 30 miles away.

As my local paper recently reported, an organization called Catalyst for Payment Reform (a coalition of big companies and the Health Care Incentives Improvement Institute) graded states on their transparency requirements regarding healthcare costs. Many states got an F; mine—Virginia—got a B, though no state agency publicizes what a given insurance company pays a given hospital.

The story made a cryptic comment that applies nationwide: It's like buying a new car without the salesman letting you know the price. Patients "often don't know how much a procedure will end up costing them until a bill arrives," the article points out.

Resources exist to help you get some idea about how much you should pay. You'll have to play Sherlock Holmes, but with an adversary worse than Professor Moriarty. There's the Medicare fee to give you a sort of price floor; then, tack on 150 percent, and you have an idea of what you should expect something to cost. To discover what Medicare pays, you'll have to...

CRACK THE INSURANCE CODE

If you have a CPT or HCPCS code, go to the Center for Medicare and Medicaid Services site at www.cms.gov/apps/physician-fee-schedule/overview.aspx. It's officially for doctors, but bear with me and I'll walk you through it.

Click on "Physician Fee Schedule Search," which takes you to a page where you have to accept the terms. You won't get much further if you don't. Then, there's a page with a "Type of Information" list; pick "Pricing Information." Below this is another list, "Select Healthcare Common Procedure Coding System," and here you pick "Single HCPCS Code." Below this is another list, "Select Carrier/Medicare Administrative Contractor (MAC) Option," and here you pick "All Carriers/MACs." Put your CPT or HCPCS code in the box, and then select "All Modifiers" from the drop-down menu.

This gives you a chart with prices that vary depending on what modifier you look at, but it provides a range of prices with a fairly narrow spread of what Medicare pays for whatever service you look up. Usually, insurance companies base the fee they pay on the Medicare payment. They mark up Medicare's amount by a certain percentage, generally around 150 percent. So, doing the same calculation gives you an idea of a reasonable fee.

There are also websites that tell you a fair price. At the risk of making you feel like a secondhand car, go to Healthcare Bluebook at www.healthcarebluebook.com. There, you can find out how much this organization thinks is a fair price. Go to the "Patient Resource" section and pick from the headings "Hospital," "Physician," "X-ray Image," "Lab," etc. Look at the drop-down menu to find the procedure you're interested in. You just need to know what category to look in; for example, an appendectomy is under "gastrointestinal" on the surgery drop-down list. If you can't find what you're looking for, submit a request for a price on whatever procedure.

This site has a lot of other useful information. You can print out forms that list the procedure and price to take to your doctor to sign, confirming the cost and creating documentation (mostly to safeguard against a billing department claiming ignorance about negotiations between you and your doctor).

The FAIR Health page at fairhealthconsumer.org/medicalcostlookup.php is another useful resource. Incidentally, this organization was established in 2009 as part of the settlement following an investigation by New York State regarding the health insurance industry's methods for determining out-of-network reimbursement. Its mission is to "bring transparency to healthcare costs." Now there's a novel idea.

This address takes you to "FH Medical Cost Lookup." Put in the relevant zip code, then indicate whether you have insurance. Enter a CPT code if you have it, or go to the drop-down list (though it's somewhat limited). Agree to the terms and get a list of procedures with their CPT codes. Click the one you want and see the "established charge." If you're looking up charges for an operation, the list includes the doctor's charge, hospital's charge, and anesthesiologist's charge, which is helpful. The downside is the list isn't comprehensive.

FAIR Health limits you to twenty searches per week for two consecutive months. These restrictions reflect the fact that the CPT code database is copyrighted by the American Medical Association (AMA). If you want to buy the whole book or e-book with all the codes, the 2014 version costs $114.95. I can't help thinking it's a bit screwy, since the information is so vital to the billing process and consumer protection.

In their magnanimity, though, the AMA gives you a single CPT code free of charge. Go to ocm.ama-assn.org/OCM/CPTRelativeValueSearch.do?submitbutton=accept. First, put in the location you're interested in, then the diagnosis. The function is very particular about your language, so talk like a doctor and be specific. "Appendix" gave me just one code for removal of the appendix and others for examination of a pathology specimen by a pathologist in the lab; when I put in "appendectomy," it came up with all the codes for the various methods of removal (laparoscopic or open).

The diagnostic related group (DRG) code tells you what a hospital charges. Look up DRGs at the HIPAA Space website at http://www.hipaaspace.com/Medical_Billing/Coding/Diagnosis_Related_Group/DRG_Code_Lookup.aspx. You contend with a massive number of variations on each major category (I put in "congestive heart failure" and it wanted to know whether it's associated with shock, pulmonary edema, renal failure, etc.). Again, use doctor-speak.

This whole business of looking up CPT codes and costs is rather complicated and technical, with sites having their own quirks making them tricky to navigate. But they're basically your only option for figuring out some of this stuff and getting an idea how much a fair price should be.

To further editorialize, besides taking issue with the fact that some of this information is copyrighted, I find it hard to believe the industry couldn't make pricing information readily accessible if they wanted to. Maybe there's just a little deliberate obfuscation?

If you're not reviewing a bill, but instead are shopping around for a procedure, make price inquiries at the offices or hospitals you're considering. In a small office-based practice, you usually speak directly to the doctor or office manager. But at a bigger practice or hospital, there's usually an accounts or billing department to speak to (in these cases, the doctor probably doesn't even know the charge for a particular procedure).

Either way, you need to know exactly what procedure you're talking about, and the right CPT or DRG code is the best way to get a reliable answer. But you may not always know, given the possible variables; if you remember my hysterectomy example from earlier, for example, it's unlikely you know how much your uterus weighs. Also, sometimes nobody knows until the time of the surgery exactly what's involved. Having your gall bladder removed laparoscopically is a very different operation and price than having it removed through a regular incision. You may start with a laparoscopic procedure, but end up needing a conventional one due to some complication.

Your insurance carrier, if you have one, has a vested interest and can be helpful in determining a good price. Then, if you want to use an out-of-network provider, ask him if he's willing to accept the insurance company's approved amount (remember, in-network doctors contractually agree to accept what the insurance pays).

Alternatively, if you don't have insurance but can find out what the doctor accepts from insurance companies for the procedure, ask if he'll accept that price from you. If you make any such special arrangement with an out-of-network provider or when you're uncovered, get the details in writing before going through with anything.

HAGGLING

Often, you can save a lot with negotiations, just like you were in some exotic Eastern bazaar. This means you have to get over any coyness about wrangling over money.

I grew up in a respectable middle-class family in England, and whenever we went to buy something, there was never any question about the price. A cup of tea was 25 pence, a newspaper cost 1 pound, and a pint of beer cost 2 quid. But when I was a med student, an ex-girlfriend working in Athens told me she could fix me up with an elective at King Paul Hospital where she worked as an orthoptist (someone who primarily treats eye movement disorders—like squints—in children).

When an old girlfriend beckons, it's hard to resist, plus it sounded like an exciting opportunity. So my friend and fellow student Blair and I booked trains across Europe. We passed the eight-hour layover in Munich in the Hofbrauhaus and were caught off guard by the strength of the German beer, cunningly sold in liters rather than mere pints. We had to be led hand in hand back to the station by a Canadian girl who fortunately knew where it was.

This elective was a bit of a joke, and involved drinking a lot of that deadly mud-like Greek coffee, but we took a week off from this punishing regimen to fly to Istanbul, "The Gateway to the East." It was like nothing we'd ever seen before.

We were awed by the cool, exotic beauty of the Blue Mosque and totally fascinated by the Grand Bazaar. This is a seething mass of humanity and glittering array of clothing, jewelry, furniture, fabrics, and trinkets of every kind. Everything is for sale, and everyone a salesman. But there are no prices.

If you want to buy something, it's a kind of game where the vendor asks some outrageous price and you counter with some trivial amount, like 15 or 20 percent of the original asking price. The more time you spend bullshitting, and the more glasses of tea (not coffee here) you drink, the better the price.

You learn not to be uncomfortable making paltry offers, despite the feigned disgust you're met with. It's a good lesson. When faced down by some intimidating billing office employee, you just haggle like it's some mustachioed, pantalooned vendor in the Grand Bazaar.

If you're dealing with a hospital, take your newfound brazenness to the accounts department. An offer of about 35 percent of the amount billed is reasonable. As noted, they don't get the chargemaster price from the insurance company. You might question the sanity of a system that bills three times what they expect to receive, but trying to explain the sanity—or lack thereof—of the system is probably neither possible nor helpful.

Also, many hospitals provide charity care or self-pay discounts, so ask about these if you're uninsured and/or in a low income bracket. This can cut down on the need for your assertive negotiator routine. Usually, a social worker or the benefits officer at the hospital is the person to talk to.

My local hospital tells me any "self-pay" gets an automatic 55 percent discount. But some might point out that 55 percent off a charge three times what it should be in the first place isn't exactly a bargain.

Many doctors who don't accept insurance (you pay them, then file a claim with your carrier) give a 20 percent discount if you pay upfront to avoid the expense and hassle of billing.

Offering to pay your entire bill upfront with cash is a powerful negotiating tool. Any businessman knows the advantages of having the money in hand as soon as possible, rather than dealing with the work, expenses, and delays of repeated billing. Also, when you don't pay and your doctor "sends you to collections" (sells your accounts receivable to a collection agency), he loses money. Incidentally, the collections agency will be a lot more obnoxious about hounding you for the money.

If you're unable to pay everything upfront, set up a payment plan. If the doctor or hospital charges interest, you may get a better rate with a loan from your bank, which also may be better than putting it on a credit card. But now we're getting into financial advice; taking it from me, or just about any doctor, would be like the Woody Allen joke about a stockbroker being someone who invests your money till it's all gone.

Again, get all the specifics of any deal you negotiate in writing and signed.

HELP WITH YOUR BILL

Patients often find this whole negotiation thing intimidating or overwhelming. Before you decide it's not for you and just shell out the full asking price, consider the help available. Start with the Patient Advocate Foundation at www.patientadvocate.org, which gives a lot of advice on agencies that help out if you're struggling. There's also a newly evolved industry of claims assistant professionals (CAPs). Something about necessity being the mother of invention springs to mind.

CAPs audit charges, find billing errors, determine proper payment, help file paperwork, challenge insurance denials, track claims, and negotiate for you. They can also help you choose the right health insurance and advise on long-term care, Medicare Part D drug plans, and other areas.

Some work on contingency, so cost nothing if they don't reduce your bill. Others charge a fixed percentage of the bill, while others charge by the hour. I've seen quoted hourly rates of $100, but even this may be a good investment if it significantly reduces a massive bill.

Brill quotes Katalin Goencz, a former hospital billing co-ordinator and member of the Alliance of Claims Assistance Professionals (ACAP). "I can pretty much always get it down 30 percent to 50 percent simply by saying the patient is ready to pay but will not pay $300 for a blood test or an X-ray."

Go to www.claims.org/refer.php to find a claims assistance professional near you. Though there's no formal certification process, ACAP says it only accepts highly experienced CAPs as members. Or, visit the Medical Billing Advocates of America at www.billadvocates.com or the CareCounsel at www.carecounsel.com, which provides a service to employers wanting to help their employees.

A debt consultation agency may be helpful in at least organizing, if not reducing, your medical bills. They should be able to help you set up a tolerable payment plan.

WANT CHEAP DRUGS?

The cost of medicine is often a significant part of healthcare expenses, and a lot of people are on a lot of drugs. There are all those harrowing stories of little old ladies having to either forgo their medicines or not eat, while the drug industry rakes in $650 billion annually. *Consumer Reports* says 90 percent of seniors rely on prescription medicines on a regular basis, but 12 percent say they've had to skip them in the past year due to price.

The cost of medicines in the U.S. are, for various reasons, a lot higher than in other countries. When North Dakota Democratic Senator Byron Dorgan was co-sponsoring an unsuccessful amendment to loosen restrictions on importing medicines into the U.S. in 2009, he pointed out that the same Nexium prescription cost $67 in France, $40 in the U.K., $37 in Germany, $36 in Spain, and $424 in the U.S., as reported in the *Washington Independent*. Unfortunately for the little guy, legislation in America tends to favor the pharmaceutical companies. Politicians, like doctors, have been manipulated by massive amounts of drug industry money.

Your doctor usually decides which medicines you're prescribed. Most patients accept that the doctor knows best and that he diligently computes all the considerations, cool as a cucumber, and prescribes you the cheapest, most effective medicine.

In your dreams.

As we've already discussed, he's probably in the pay of a conniving drug company, schmoozed, wined, dined, and flirted with by some coquettish drug rep, and he just happens to think the company's newest name-brand antihypertensive is vastly superior to anything else available. And even if he resists these influences, there are numerous others at work on his prescription decision-making process.

Most health insurance plans cover medicines. But there are usually different tiers of coverage, and you may have to pay a higher co-pay for medicines in tier 3 than those in tier 1; the difference can be as extreme as $10 for one and $150 for another. The exact amount varies by plan, not all carriers use the same tier structures, and drugs can change tiers. It's enough to bring you to tears.

Sometimes, really expensive drugs aren't covered at all. Or, they have to be pre-authorized by the insurance, which can be a major pain for the doctor.

Getting your insurance company's formulary and paying attention to the tiers is worthwhile, as is getting your doctor to pay attention, too. As with tests, doctors generally have no idea what medicines cost. Most carriers' formularies have medicine from each treatment group in tier 1 that does pretty much the same job as some of the more expensive medicines; ask your doctor about viable tier 1 alternatives if he's prescribing something pricey.

Now I'll walk you through a few ways of getting cheaper drugs.

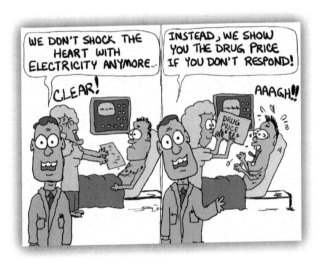

OPTION 1: GENERICS

If you take an expensive name-brand medicine, you and your doctor can probably find a cheaper alternative, provided your doctor hasn't been completely won over by the reps. Name-brand medicines are the most expensive and profitable for the drug company, so they are vigorously promoted.

There's often a generic version—it's the same active ingredient—of what you take, provided the drug isn't still protected by patent. Some people are nervous about taking generics, but this is baseless worry. Ask your doctor about a generic alternative. But even these can be expensive, especially in their first year, when one manufacturer has an exclusive contract.

After the first year of generic availability, the market opens up and prices drop. From here on, the cost differences between name-brand and generic is typically significant. Public Citizen's website Worst Pills, Best Pills (www.worstpills.org) offers a glimpse. For example, if you have asthma, generic albuterol is 52.3 percent cheaper than name-brand Ventolin; if you have high blood pressure, generic lisinopril is 47.1 percent cheaper than brand-name Prinivil; and generic fluid pill furosemide is 47.1 percent cheaper than brand-name Lasix. *Consumer Reports* notes if you don't have insurance, one month's supply of generic cholesterol medicine simvastatin (20 mg) costs $70, whereas the name-brand version of the same, Zocor, costs $175; $42 to $84 of brand-name Glucotrol (10 mg) for diabetes can be had in generic form as glipizide for $4 to $8.

If what you take is still protected by its twenty-year patent, there's no exact generic equivalent. Often, though, there's a very similar generic alternative. For example, Micardis (the brand name of telmisartan) is a blood pressure medicine in the angiotensin receptor blocker (ARB) class. Its patent just expired in 2014. While it was protected, though, lots of other similar, but not identical, ARB-class medicines were available as generics, like valsartan (brand name Diovan), irbesartan (Avapro), olmesartan (Benicar), and losartan (Cozaar). In many instances, these could be used to do the same job.

Or, another name-brand product may be cheaper if it's been around longer. For example, another class of medicines for hypertension, angiotensin-converting enzyme (ACE) inhibitors (like generic lisinopril and brand-name Zestril and Prinivil), have been out longer than the very similar ARBs, so they're cheaper.

Pharmaceutical companies also come up with tricks to extend their patents on name-brand medicines. When you're aware of these, it often opens up cheaper options. Manufacturers frequently devise some kind of fancy new delivery system for their drug, or they turn it into a combination medicine.

For example, your name-brand medicine may be patent-protected in its new slow- or extended-release version. Lots of these medicines are available in generic form if you take them a little more frequently in an older standard form. You sacrifice a little convenience, but can save considerable sums.

Consider Coreg CR. Carvedilol, a beta blocker for treating hypertension and heart disease, is its active ingredient. Coreg CR is time-released for a once-daily dose, while you have to take generic carvedilol twice per day. But a standard Coreg CR prescription is $141.99 for thirty pills ($4.73 per pill), whereas thirty twice-daily generic carvedilol pills are only $14.99 (50 cents per pill); it's only half the supply, but it's still way cheaper.

The other fandangle is to mix together two medicines available as generics and patent the combo. The blood pressure medicine Exforge, for example, is a combination of amlodipine and valsartan; the diabetes medicine Janumet is sitagliptin and metformin. You might reduce your expenditure by getting the two generic components separately.

Mind you, this can work the other way around. Sometimes, a combination medicine is cheaper than its components separately. Lisinopril-hydrochlorthiazide is a combination of two blood pressure medicines. Filling prescriptions for the two separately is likely to cost more.

Option 2: Over The Counter

Occasionally, you can get away with over-the-counter (OTC) medicines (see *Medical Kit* for advice on what's treatable with OTCs), and they are often cheaper. In particular, store brands at big chains are usually the cheapest OTC options.

Employing my best investigative journalism chops, I nosed around a little at Wegmans and Walmart for comparisons. At Wegmans, name-brand Advil costs $8.59 for 100 pills, but the store's own Top Care brand cost $2.49 for 100 pills of the same dosage. Name-brand OTC Zyrtec costs $17.99 for 100 pills, but the equivalent All Day Allergy costs only $5.99.

In Walmart, a 4-ounce bottle of Robitussin DM costs $5.64, but the same quantity of store-brand Tussin costs $1.96; baby aspirin (81 mg) from Bayer costs $9.47 for 200 pills, but $0.98

for 100 of the store brand's; Prilosec (20.6 mg) runs $9.94 for fourteen pills, versus $6.97 for fourteen generic omeprazole.

To see if there's an OTC equivalent to your prescription (which is admittedly not common), check out the FDA's "Orange Book" at www.accessdata.fda.gov/scripts/cder/ob/default.cfm.

Don't forget to look for generic equivalents of name-brand OTC medicines, too. Just compare the active ingredient(s) and quantities in the name-brand to the store-brand and other generics nearby on the shelf.

OPTION 3: THE CHEAPEST STORE

It may sound obvious, but not everybody bothers to shop around to fill a prescription. Considerable savings may be found by choosing the right place to buy, especially in the long run. There's no one right answer for everyone, of course. A lot depends on what stores are convenient for you and which drugs you take.

"Wally World" (Walmart) and Target both have $4 medicine lists. These are comprised of hundreds of generic and OTC medicines, all sold for $4. Giant and other supermarkets have similar lists, while Publix, Wegmans, and other supermarkets offer a number of generic antibiotics for free.

Walgreens has its own $4 list, but there's an annual fee to take advantage of the program. It's $35 for a family or $20 for an individual, and you are ineligible if you have Medicare or

Medicaid. Many other stores charge a base fee that opens up access to cheaper medicines, too.

Whether it's worth paying a fee to get discounts depends on a few factors. Stores have different eligibility requirements, so first find out if you qualify. If it's a store-wide loyalty card, confirm that it's honored in the pharmacy (it isn't always), and that the drugs you take are covered (not all of them always are). Then it's just a matter of math. How much is the annual fee and what percentage does it save you on your pharmacy purchases? Convert the percentages to dollars for what you buy over the course of a year, and if it adds up to more than the fee, it's worthwhile.

Print out the $4 list from your store of choice and bring it to your appointment. Let your doctor look it over to see whether you can take something on it.

Beyond these $4 lists, of the brick-and-mortar pharmacies in my area, the one in the discount club Costco seems to be the cheapest. They reputedly use cheap drugs as a "loss leader" to entice customers into the store, though you don't have to be a paying member to use the pharmacy. I found the best price for my contact lenses at another discount club, BJ's, where the wife and I are members.

OPTION 4: BUY ONLINE

Usually, the best prices are online. Options include the websites of brick-and-mortar stores like the ones I'm talking about here, or online-only pharmacies. Some are U.S.-based, but the lowest prices tend to be from international pharmacies, many in Canada. One thing to watch out for, though: the medicine might be cheap, but the shipping costs can be exorbitant.

A lot of people are nervous about buying drugs online, and there are good reasons to be. But with some precautions, it opens up a world of savings possibilities.

Know going in, there are lots of fly-by-night websites that will rip you off.

For example, the FDA site tells of ordering anti-flu medicine Tamiflu (oseltamivir) online as part of a surveillance operation. The ordered arrived "in an unmarked envelope with a postmark from India" and consisted of unlabeled white tablets that "were found to contain talc and acetaminophen (the ingredient in Tylenol), but none of the active ingredient oseltamivir."

The FDA says the best way to get safe, predictable, properly stored and shipped medicines is to buy only from U.S.-based pharmacies. Then, only use those with pharmacists available for consulting and that require a prescription, rather than those that don't require a prescription or offer a virtual consultation for their doctors to write you one.

A further safeguard is to only use sites approved by the National Association of Boards of Pharmacies. Sites approved by NABP are issued a verified internet pharmacy practice site (VIPPS) certification, indicated by a lozenge-shaped logo on the site, which you can click to confirm authenticity.

You may be tempted by low prices to use pharmacies outside the U.S. First, importing medicines from overseas by mail or in person is illegal. But if it's not something dangerous and is clearly just for personal use, the FDA, in its benevolence, turns a blind eye. Still, there's no saying when it might decide to enforce the law.

The FDA is a little overprotective, some say. Its guidelines exclude Canadian pharmacies. A lot of people go to Canada, either in person on one of these modern-day pilgrimages in which masses of geriatrics maraud across the border by the busload, or via the internet.

Many claim Canadian sites are safe, especially if you look for those certified by the Canadian International Pharmacy Association, which issues verification in the form of the CIPA seal.

Lest you think this Canadian regulatory body is just a bunch of yahoos, a respectable U.S. agency, the National Bureau of Economic Research, took a look and "confirms that medications sold online by pharmacies accredited by the CIPA are 100 percent authentic."

All in all, the objections raised by the FDA and NABP about medicines from Canada are usually about trivial stuff, like that packaging and labeling don't comply with FDA standards.

To compare online pharmacy prices, go to www.eDrug-Search.com or www.Pharmacychecker.com. But in my experience, things get harder after you find a good price on one of these sites. I found maneuvering around the pharmacy sites themselves difficult. I couldn't get past the "useful" information and promotions (though that's my complaint about almost all websites these days). Also, they all seem to insist you sign up before you can get more information. My fear is that once I provide my email address, my inbox will become as engorged as all the Viagra, Levitra, and Cialis spam suggest my phallus should be.

Some websites are also helpful for showing you alternatives to your prescription. If you search for your drug on the CVS site at www.cvs.com/drug, for example, there's an option to see class-related drugs. The AARP website has a similar feature at drugsavings.aarp.org/Default.aspx. There's also Epocrates and its mobile apps, which I've mentioned before, at www.epocrates.com.

OPTION 5: MEDICARE PART D

This one's just for the old folks with Medicare. Basic Medicare doesn't pay for medicines, so for drug coverage, you need Part D. There are all different plans with all different benefits offered by all different vendors, and it can be tricky deciding how much coverage to get. A lot depends on which medicines you take, how much they cost, and how long you'll be on them.

In line with its effort to help us old buggers with our healthcare expenses, the American Association of Retired Persons (AARP, of which I am a proud card-carrying member) publishes www.aarp.org/health/medicare-insurance/medicare_partD_ guide to help you choose the best plan. Or, try www.medicare.gov itself and plug in your prescriptions.

Take into account the infamous "doughnut hole," though. After you and your part D insurance together have paid a certain amount (it was $2,970 in 2013), you have to pay 50 percent of the cost of name-brand drugs and 86 percent of the cost of generic drugs until you reach the "catastrophic coverage" limit ($4,750 in 2013), after which you only have to pay 5 percent of the cost of your prescriptions.

You might be forgiven for wondering who could have dreamed up such a complicated plan. The government, of course. The good news is, the doughnut hole will be gradually phased out—on a very complicated schedule—by the ACA.

For those with very low income, there's the so-called "Extra Help" Medicare plan. With this, you're exempted from the coverage gap/doughnut hole. Again, there's a lot to look into. Your pharmacist, an oft-neglected source of information, may be able to help advise you about plans.

OPTION 6: PATIENT ASSISTANCE PROGRAMS (PAP s)

If you're really struggling to afford your medicines, some pharmaceutical companies offer discounted or free drugs through patient assistance programs, sometimes in the form of drug discount cards. It's gracious of them, though they can afford it. Accessing these programs, however, is no cakewalk.

The Federal Trade Commission (FTC) blithely suggests asking your physician for help with your application. But, dare I suggest, your doctor may not know how to navigate this maze any better than you, and may not be too thrilled to spend his time trying to figure it out.

Companies, like the SelectCare Benefits Network (http://www.scbn.org), have even sprung up to help with the application process, which can be complicated. SCBN gives dire warnings that the 250-odd assistance programs "have evolved into large bureaucracies with long complicated enrollment processes that can overwhelm patients and discourage participation." Paperwork is complicated and has to be submitted every three months, they say, and "a program will often reject a patient for a single error in the paperwork."

Of course, these companies stand to benefit from hyping the horrors of the PAP application process. Some attack these companies for taking advantage of those who can least afford it. ABC News did an exposé on this very topic, and it seems these companies are exaggerating the difficulty of applying to discourage people from applying on their own.

ABC's recommendation—and that of the FTC—is to go to Partnership for Prescription Assistance, a sort of clearinghouse run by Big Pharma. With some personal information about your medicines, the site directs you to a suitable assistance program for your needs at no charge. Find it at www.pparx.org.

If you qualify, a PAP can save you a lot of money. Most programs have the same basic eligibility requirements. You must:

- Be a U.S. resident
- Not have any kind of insurance that covers medicine

- Have an income low enough that paying for your medicines would be a hardship, which typically means an income not exceeding 200 percent of the Federal Poverty Guidelines (which, in 2015, works out to $23,540 for a single individual or $48,500 for a family of four)

Medicare has a low-income subsidy program to help pay premiums, annual deductibles, drug co-payments, and coinsurance if your financial assets are small enough. As of this writing, you must have assets totaling less than $13,440 if you're single or $26,860 if you're married. Application is through Social Security, and can be completed online at www.socialsecurity.gov/medicare/prescriptionhelp/.

Various other organizations give assistance with prescription costs (and with medical costs in general). A few examples include Chronic Disease Fund, Family Wize, Healthwell Foundation, and NeedyMeds. There's a good list compiled by Martine Ehrenclou, M.A., in *The Take-Charge Patient: How YOU Can Get the Best Medical Care*.

OTHER OPTIONS FOR SAVING ON MEDICINES
Cut Them in Half

Getting a stronger pill and halving it is a potential money-saver. This is easy if the pill is scored, or get a pill cutter. A 1000 mg metformin pill for diabetes doesn't magically accomplish anything two 500 mg pills don't. If you're on 500 mg a day, you get two months' worth out of a one-month supply of 1000 mg tablets. Ask your doctor if there's a stronger pill you can do this with.

There is one proviso, however. If the pill has a special coating or delivery system (which is liable to make it more expensive, incidentally) you can't cut it or break it up. Ask your doctor or pharmacist whether it's safe to cut a pill beforehand.

Don't Throw Them Away

Save on medicines by not throwing them out. This is a bit controversial, as everyone's urged to clear out their medicine cabinets and throw out anything the instant it reaches its expiry date. There's anxiety about expiration dates—or irrational hysteria, if you ask me (talking as a parsimonist).

Manufacturers are required by law to label an expiry date. It's the date before which they guarantee 100 percent efficacy and safety. But that doesn't mean the medicine is unsafe or ineffective right afterward. In fact, a study commissioned by the military—distressed at the prospect of throwing out huge quantities of expired drugs—found 90 percent of more than 100 prescription and OTC drugs were "perfectly good to use even 15 years after the expiration date."

Admittedly, these medicines were kept in their original containers under ideal temperature and humidity conditions. And there are a few medicines, like liquid antibiotics, nitroglycerine, and insulin, which do not have a long shelf life. But providing you are not taking medicines for something too crucial (like anti-seizure or heart medicine), you're probably

OK taking medicines significantly past their expiry date. I do.

Ask your pharmacist for specific advice. But bear in mind that pharmacists—like many others in healthcare and other walks of life these days—tend to be cautious and risk-averse, and are probably reluctant to tell you, "Oh, sure, it's probably OK to take, even though it's ten years past its expiration date." Plus, they probably would prefer to sell you more new drugs.

Take Samples. Maybe. For a Little While.

Not infrequently, your doctor gives you samples of something from his pharmaceutical cabinet. We had a large, well-stocked cabinet in my office. When I'd fling open the doors, revealing all those shelves brimming with boxes and bottles to find some sample of the latest, greatest medicine, patients would sometimes practically orgasm.

Contrary to what some of the more drug-crazed patients seemed to think, the samples aren't exciting psychotropics and narcotics. But they are a bit of a Trojan horse.

An analysis in *Medical Care* (April 2008) noted, "Individuals receiving samples have higher prescription expenditures than their counterparts," and are "disproportionately burdened by prescription costs even after sample receipt."

Samples, of course, are of the newest name-brand products (and therefore almost always the most expensive) the drug company is actively pushing. You might get free medicine for a week or a month, but after that you're paying through the nose.

One saving grace is when your doctor uses samples to test you on a kind of medicine, then writes you a prescription for a generic equivalent or older version. This is definitely considered "not cricket" by the drug reps, not that most of them know what cricket is, I'd guess. Or, occasionally, a doctor may schmooze the drug rep to scratch together enough samples to keep a particularly needy patient (or one who knows something particularly compromising about the doctor) supplied on an ongoing basis.

FALLING INTO THE SAFETY NET

A "safety net" of various health clinics provides cheap and sometimes free care. There are about 9,000 state and federally supported Community Health Clinics serving low-income and rural populations. There are also Federally Qualified Health Clinics that usually charge on an income-dependent sliding fee scale.

A nationwide network of some 1,300 free clinics provides an estimated two to three and a half million medical and dental appointments annually. The Lloyd Moss Free Clinic in Fredericksburg, of which I am currently the medical director, is one. These clinics are supported by charitable donations and mostly staffed by volunteers. Jennifer Depaul, writing in the *Fiscal Times*, suggests these "just might be one of America's best kept health secrets."

The free clinic showcases a Catch-22 of the American health-care system. So many of the patients lost their jobs because they got sick, and thus lost their health insurance right when they needed it most. Fortunately, it looks like this will change with the ACA.

As for eligibility, the free clinics require patients have no insurance and little income; they commonly use 200 percent of the Federal Poverty Guidelines as the cutoff. Many of these establishments have struggled in the recent economic slowdown. "Patient demand for free and charitable clinics was up 40 percent in 2011, but donations were down 20 percent," notes Nicole Lamoureux, executive director of the National Association of Free and Charitable Clinics (NAFC).

To find a free clinic near you, visit the NAFC site at http://www.nafcclinics.org/clinics/search.

FURTHER HELP WITH PAYING YOUR BILLS

There are a number of places to turn—including government programs, charities, and various organizations and associations—that provide financial assistance and other support for people in need.

The Children's Health Insurance Program provides State and Federal funds to families that don't qualify for Medicaid who are struggling with medical bills due to a child's care. Go to www.insurekidsnow.gov/state/index.html for more information on the program and enrollment.

The Patient Advocacy Foundation (www.patientadvocate.org) helps coordinate between patients, insurers, and employers and provides a lot of helpful information about healthcare. Go to its National Financial Resource Directory under the site's Resources drop-down menu to search for aid possibilities.

Medical Debt Help is another good resource, which says it can reduce your medical bills; go to www.debt.org/medical-debt-help.

Another smart step is to contact the national, state, or local office of any relevant injury- or disease-specific organization.

"Crowd funding" is a modern-age way to collect charitable donations to help you out with medical bills. Basically, you use a social media network to solicit donations. GiveForward (www.giveforward.com) is one site set up for this purpose.

As a last resort, you can join the 60 percent forced into bankruptcy by their medical bills.

DYING IS EXPENSIVE

Some of the worst value for the money comes at the end of life, often for futile care. "We end up spending about one-third of our overall healthcare resources in the last year of life," says Dr. Jonathan Bergman of the University of California in Los Angeles. He's one of the authors of a study about healthcare costs for terminal care, published in the *Archives of Internal Medicine* in October 2010. And, each year, Medicare spends more than $50 billion on patients for their last two months of life, reports *60 Minutes.*

I mention it here because it's such a significant healthcare cost. But I've covered end-of-life care—and how to cut down on what you spend on it—in great detail in the next chapter.

CHAPTER 6

GETTING THE RIGHT DEATH

———◆———

THE RIGHT DEATH?

PERHAPS IT SOUNDS A LITTLE weird and morbid. But the medical profession is surprisingly bad at dealing with dying and end-of-life stuff, and many patients suffer unnecessarily because of it. Countless families stress and grieve more than they should, plus they are often left with huge bills as a bitter legacy of their loved one.

Of the approximately two and a half million deaths per year in the U.S., only 10 percent are sudden deaths, notes *The New York Times* columnist Jane Brody in her excellent book *Jane Brody's Guide to the Great Beyond* (which has lots of useful information beyond what I can include here). "That leaves more than two million people who die of protracted illness," she says. This means a great deal of end-of-life care.

As bioethics research organization The Hastings Center puts it, "Death is an inevitable aspect of the human condition. Dying badly is not."

A WORD ON TERMINOLOGY

On a point of terminology, the term "loved one" always puts me in mind of Evelyn Waugh's wickedly satirical novel of the same name, based around the fictional funeral home Whispering Glades. But it's convenient shorthand for relatives, partners, and close friends, so I'll use it despite its cheesiness.

I should probably clarify exactly what I'm talking about in this chapter. "Death" is fairly self-explanatory, but terminal care is usually thought of as the last few days to the last few weeks before a person dies. But really it can—and as I get into below, often should—come into the picture much earlier on in the illness.

The phrase "terminal care" may bring cancer to mind, with its harrowing course of multiple rounds of treatment and inexorable, rapid downhill slide. But approximately 50 percent of hospice care (care for the dying) is for non-cancer patients, notes Gail Gazelle, M.D. of Boston's Brigham and Women's Hospital in *The New England Journal of Medicine*.

Usually, these others are people whose various vital organs are pooping out. Kidney or liver failure, congestive heart failure, dementia, and COPD are common examples. The decline may be less linear and more protracted than with cancer, as the patient is "circling the drain," as one brusque pulmonologist described the progress of one dear old lady patient with terminal emphysema we shared.

DYING THEN VS. NOW

As with many facets of medical care, advances in medical technology have had profound effects on the business of dying.

In the old days, dying was like experiencing bad weather, as end-of-life researcher Joanne Lynn puts it; it "strikes without warning, and you get through it or you don't."

People used to be more accepting, chalking death up to the will of a higher power. They prepared themselves for the inevitable by studying guides like *Ars Moriendi* (*The Art of Dying*), a popular work published in many languages in the 1400s when the Black Death was annihilating large portions of the population. It offers protocols and procedures for a good death. It instructs the reader on not succumbing to lack of faith, despair, impatience, spiritual pride, or avarice and how to ensure your place in heaven by cozying up to Jesus.

But now, innovations and "progress" mean we have to constantly make choices. The advent of stuff like ventilators, pacemakers, dialysis, antibiotics, chemotherapy, radiotherapy, and artificial feeding extends and complicates things.

Or, as surgeon and journalist Atul Gawande puts it in his great article on terminal care in the August 2010 *The New Yorker*, "We imagine that we can wait until the doctors tell us that there is nothing more they can do." But rarely is the toolbox empty. "Rarely is there *nothing* more that doctors can do."

Having all those clever interventions makes it hard for enthusiastic doctors to restrain themselves. Consider the case of Bert Keizer's dad.

As I was writing this, I came across what seemed to me a description of a typically horrendous end-of-life scenario involving a "cascade" of mindless interventions. It was written by Keizer, another writer/doctor hybrid who holds a degree in philosophy, works in a nursing home in Amsterdam, and whose best-known book is *Dancing with Mr. D*. It was written in Dutch, then translated by Keizer himself.

I include the description verbatim. In May 1994,

"My father was 87 years old, a dedicated smoker of roll-ups all his life, and in recent years increasingly short of breath on account of emphysema.

One of the most ill-starred meetings in modern medicine is between a frail defenseless old man nearing the end of his life, and an agile young intern at the beginning of his career.

Soon after my father's admission to hospital, chest X-rays were taken, and he was seen by a chest physician. He prescribed oxygen, mucolytics, antibiotics and physiotherapy. My father did not improve. A pulmonary embolus could not with all certainty be excluded so he was put on anticoagulants. He was very feverish and anxious, and at night he was delirious.

The doctor suspected an element of cardiac failure, so he called in the cardiologist. After another set of X-rays and an ECG had duly been performed, this colleague added diuretics to the medication and went on his way. The patient however did not improve at all; on the contrary he seemed to be slipping away from us.

On his sixth day in hospital he passed a bloody stool, probably caused by impacted faecal matter damaging the intestinal mucosa on its way out. Now the gastroenterologist was called in. Of course he advised a colonoscopy to exclude the possibility of cancer. In order for the colonoscopy to be possible my father was given about the same amount of purgative as Lord Byron had had to sustain [a reference to the death of Byron from his doctor's insistence on repeated bleedings, which Keizer relates earlier], and on the evening before the procedure my mother found him drenched in his own mess. He had totally lost his bearings at this stage and was restless at night, trying to climb out of bed forgetting he had a catheter. In order to prevent these hazardous nocturnal excursions, he was given a tranquilizer, haloperidol.

On the seventh day he could hardly speak because of the tremor caused by the haloperidol, which made him all shaky and tremulous. He was taken for a colonoscopy nevertheless, and the doctor found a polyp in his colon, which he proceeded to remove with a cauterizer, almost burning a hole in the intestinal wall, as he told me excitedly later, and certainly causing considerable blood loss

On the ninth day one of the nurses came up with the suggestion that my father was probably an Alzheimer's patient. The thought being, if there was a thought behind this suggestion, that if they mutter incomprehensibly, they're probably demented. A psychiatrist and a neurologist were called in to evaluate this possibility, a brain scan was arranged and admission to a nursing home was put on the agenda.

He had hardly been eating and was laying passively in bed, and now severe bedsores were threatening. In order to do something about this, the dermatologist was called in. During these ten days my father had been seen by an internist consultant, a pulmonary physician, a cardiologist, a gastroenterologist, a psychiatrist, a neurologist and a dermatologist. He had been subject to four X-rays, uncomfortable but not unsettling, many blood tests and the gruesome procedure of bowel cleaning prior to the colonoscopy. Even if he had not been feverish and sedated he would have been completely baffled after so many encounters.

The net outcome of all this high-flown medical expertise was that he had turned from a very ill old man into a physical and mental wreck with whom it was almost impossible to communicate. When, to top it all, the consultant wanted to call a nephrologist because of a touch of renal failure that was now showing up in his blood tests, we finally called a halt to all this and asked his GP to intervene.

The family doctor put in his dentures, then looked for and thoroughly cleaned his glasses, and after a lot of fumbling managed to get his hearing aid properly positioned. He then sat down with him and spoke for about half an hour. When asked what he really wanted, my father said he wanted to be left alone to die in peace. He was moved to a geriatric ward in a neighboring hospital, was given some morphine, and died peacefully three days later. A week after his death the pathologist called me to report the benignant aspect of the polyp removed."

Though this is from a few years back and outside the U.S., it's a classic story of what happens to patients when the machine gets rolling. In the U.S. in this day and age, this guy would quite likely undergo even more tests and procedures, and probably more sophisticated and more expensive ones.

There are endless examples of this kind of thing. In her book *The Cost of Hope: A Memoir*, Amanda Bennett complains about her husband's last few weeks of life.

"He had his blood drawn eight times, urine collected at least twice. There was a CT scan of his chest and an MRI of his brain. A physical therapist dropped by several times. A nutritionist talked about cancer fatigue, decompensating, and calorie needs. Over the stay, at least 29 professionals—nurses, physical therapists, a nutritionist, and nine M.D.s—attended to his needs. We had never met any of them before, and I don't recall ever meeting the majority of them even then." She complains how "different sick body parts are treated one after the other" in a dysfunctional system "that feels like a conveyor belt."

In his *The New Yorker* piece, Gawande describes a visit to an intensive care unit where the critical care physician on duty said she was "running a warehouse for the dying." Out of the ten patients in the unit, only two were likely to leave the hospital for any length of time. Typical was an almost 80-year-old woman at the end of her life, with irreversible congestive heart failure, who was in the ICU for the second time in three weeks, drugged to oblivion and tubed in most natural orifices and a few artificial ones. There was the 70-year-old with a cancer that had metastasized to her lungs and bone who had a fungal pneumonia (that arises only in the final phase of the illness). She had chosen to forgo treatment, but her oncologist pushed her to change her mind, and she was put on a ventilator and antibiotics.

Another woman, in her 80s and with end-stage respiratory and kidney failure, had been in the unit for two weeks. Her husband had died after a long illness, with a feeding tube and a tracheotomy, and she had mentioned that she didn't want to die that way. But her children couldn't let her go, and asked to proceed with the placement of various devices, including a permanent tracheotomy, a feeding tube, and a dialysis catheter. "So now she just lay there tethered to her pumps, drifting in and out of consciousness."

This futile care is not just a form of torture for patients, but it takes a toll on the staff as well. I recently came across a lament in a medical blog's comment stream, which I include in part and unedited:

"As an ICU Nurse, I realize that I have a choice to work where I do. However, the torture I exact on my sick and dying patients is not justifiable just because it is available. Last week I took care of a 73 year old woman who was incapable of speaking, eating, moving, whose only capacity to communicate with me was to moan. She of course, did not have an advance directive, so this end stage renal diseased post CVA fellow human being is being dialyzed, with no possible hope of return to a reasonably healthy state. I routinely ask forgiveness from my patients before I turn them to change their dressings on their bedsores, try to start yet another central line, or inject them with a 3x a week shot of procrit, at mere thousands per injection."

The commenter condemns the "ruthless system," saying she prays "I never hold the view from the bed."

It may sound like I'm condemning intensive care, which is not exactly the case. The ICU isn't a good place for terminal care. What I condemn is when things are done simply because they can be. When a doctor can think of things to do—a CT of the abdomen with abdominal pain, an MRI of the head in mental status change, a feeding tube if a patient can't eat, a ventilator if he can't breathe—they tend to be ordered, even if they have no bearing on the big picture.

This culture dominates the ICU. Doing something rather than nothing is the default position, unless someone has said no through an advance directive (which I'll get to soon). And so the ICU is often the wrong place for a dying patient.

But all too often, they end up in the ICU or some other acute care setting. There are a billion interventions available. They're doable, and, to be cynical, they're billable.

So, it's common for people to spend the last days of their lives in pain, confused, sedated or restrained, with a tube in every orifice, on a ventilator, unable to talk or have any meaningful interactions. Visits are constantly interrupted by tests, treatments, nurses, doctors, and therapists.

If this is a necessary evil to buy more time—if quantity rather than quality is what you're looking for—so be it. But a 1998 study by the nonprofit Bureau of Economic Research found neither high spending nor more days in the hospital have much to do with how long a patient lived.

The Coping with Cancer Project and the Dartmouth Atlas Project looked at discrepancies in distribution of healthcare resources. In the latter, Dr. Elliott Fisher, a professor at Dartmouth University's Geisel School of Medicine, noted that terminally ill cancer patients who received CPR or were admitted near death to intensive care did not live longer. And, incidentally, they had a substantially worse quality of life (which is not hard to believe).

The usefulness of ICUs in terminal care isn't just questionable for patients. Dr. Joan Teno, a researcher from Brown University involved in the Coping with Cancer Project, reported that six months after patients who had CPR or were admitted to the ICU had died, their caregivers were three times as likely to suffer major depression. It seems the more intensive care a patient receives, the more the family feels the patient was not well cared for, she says.

Recognition of the tendency to wildly over-treat has become a focus of the profession's penchant for cynicism and black humor (which, in defense of my colleagues, is something of a coping mechanism against the freaky stuff we deal with). Bennett recounts the hospital chaplain telling her a joke circulating among the staff about an orderly going to the morgue to retrieve a dead body who instead finds a note that reads, "Gone to X-ray."

WHY IS DEATH SUCH A MESSY BUSINESS?

Multiple factors account for why terminal patients are treated this way, with this unthinking insistence on doing everything.

It's hard for enthusiastic doctors to restrain themselves and not use all those tools in the toolbox. "The system in this country requires us to ask permission *not* to do a treatment," writes chaplain, author, and speaker Hank Dunn in his book *Hard Choices for Loving People*. Doing is the default, often without consideration for the big picture. This is what leads to a lot of dying badly.

"Avoidance and denial" are cultural hallmarks when it comes to death, notes Brody. Difficulty dealing with the end of life is found "among physicians as well as lay people," she says.

Like other human beings, doctors are uncomfortable dealing with death. Telling someone they have some incurable fatal disease is not a subject that makes for an enjoyable chat like you might have over a beer or cup of coffee.

This discomfort with death is partly inculcated in medical school.

Maybe it's inevitable that medical students carry the philosophies and prejudices learned in med school with them into maturity and fully plumed doctorhood. They're trained to save lives at all cost and to consider it a blow to their ego when their patients die. "Patients' deaths, for many doctors, represent a kind of failure," writes Pauline Chen, M.D., surgeon and author of *Final Exam: A Surgeon's Reflections on Mortality.*

The deficiency in death education motivated the person whose name is probably most associated with dealing with dying patients: Elisabeth Kübler-Ross.

She was an instructor at the University of Chicago's medical school who worked with terminally ill patients. Critical of how the curriculum failed to address this aspect of healthcare, she wrote the acclaimed book *On Death and Dying,* published in 1969.

Kübler-Ross is particularly famous for describing the five stages of reactions of someone diagnosed with a deadly disease—denial, anger, bargaining, depression, and acceptance. Of course, there may be nuances like resentment or frustration as manifestations of anger, and people may jump backward and forward between the stages.

"There's an overall pattern of how humans deal with forthcoming death," says Sherri McCarthy, a psychology professor at Northern Arizona University and grief counselor. "Shock or denial is a pretty universal first reaction," she explains. Patients often say things like, "It's a mistake" or "I'll see a different doctor."

Doctors can go through a similar string of responses, but often mixed with guilt at not having prevented a patient from developing a fatal illness or dying.

The lack in doctors' know-how and their discomfort dealing with death and dying has been recognized in some circles, and attempts have been made to get a better handle on it. With its clever, if not slightly contrived, acronym, the Study to Understand Prognosis and Preferences for Outcomes and Risk of Treatment (SUPPORT) trial was a four-year study conducted in five university hospitals starting in 1989. It "revealed a profound lack of awareness of the needs of the terminally ill," reports Brody, and the majority of doctors had no idea what patients wanted regarding resuscitation.

As a result, "Many of these patients experienced prolonged deaths while being treated with costly, invasive life-sustaining technology and spent the last days in an intensive care unit, all but cut off from their family and friends," she says. "Half the hospitalized patients who were conscious at the end of life suffered moderate to severe pain at least half the time."

"Even more disturbing," she reports that the authors noted, "after two years of active intervention by specially trained nurses who served as liaison between patients and their families and between patients, physicians and hospital staff, there was no noticeable improvement."

Some are trying to address this. The University of Iowa Carver College of Medicine has an end-of-life-care course to help students become aware of their attitudes by discussing and writing about how they see their own deaths happening and about prior experiences with death. It's hoped this will help them face concerns about losing composure, about helplessness, and about pain and personal grief.

The American Academy of Family Physicians encourages preparation of doctors in training with a policy saying residents "should demonstrate attitudes that encompass the ability to compassionately and empathetically deliver bad news."

Chen notes many attending physicians teaching med students and new doctors have their own hang-ups about dealing with death. They tend to lack insight into how their deficiencies get passed on to those they teach.

I suspect the new fashion for doctors to forgo caring for their own patients in the hospital, leaving the work instead to hospitalists, is another factor behind the don't-look-at-the-big-picture-and-do-everything system of dealing with terminal patients.

Hospitalists are often young, and therefore still more strongly indoctrinated and usually enthusiastic about all the interventions available. When a technology exists, it's particularly hard for them not to use it as a knee-jerk reaction. A mental status change automatically calls for a CT or MRI scan; a GI bleed buys a colonoscopy, with all its attendant morbidity and costs; blocked coronary arteries tend to equal a coronary artery bypass graft (CABG), at least to a cardiac surgeon ("To a man with a hammer, everything looks like a nail"); poor food intake and bang, in with a feeding tube; and so on.

The big picture matters. If a patient is about to die of cancer, there's no good reason to perform a colonoscopy. If a patient is about to die of kidney failure, there's no good reason to do a CABG.

And, dare I say it, decisions are sometimes influenced by the doctor's vested interests. To be charitable, many interventions are employed because the doctor has seen them used to great effect in non-end-of-life situations. To be cynical, tests, imaging, chemotherapy, surgery, and all that ICU stuff is well reimbursed, so there's financial incentive.

Hospitalists also generally don't have a lot of primary care experience, nor a longstanding personal relationship with patients and their families. This means they aren't in a good position to know their wants or to comfortably have one of those "game plan" conversations.

Keizer describes "one of the most ill-starred meetings" as taking place between his dad, "a frail defenseless old man" and "an agile young intern at the beginning of his career."

This intervention obsession is even reflected in medical jokes, as with the concept of "a Harvard death." That's when the doctor has so skillfully controlled the patient's fluid input and output that their blood chemistry and electrolytes are perfectly within normal ranges, but the cussed patient up and dies.

As another obstacle to a good death, alternative medicines can generate over-enthusiasm when hope wanes.

Sometimes, extravagant claims are made for complementary and alternative treatments, and desperate patients may grasp at them. But if these alternative treatments were as effective as some of the promoters claim, every oncologist would be using them; they don't have so much antipathy toward CAM practitioners that they would forgo an effective treatment. Be on guard against people with offbeat treatments they insist provide a cure.

CURING VS. MANAGING ILLNESS

Before getting deeper into end-of-life planning, it's helpful to know what your options are. Often, they come down to the choice between definitive care and palliative care.

Definitive care means doing everything to try to eradicate the illness. It seeks to cure the cancer, for example, or to get the heart, lungs, liver, or kidneys working normally again or find some workable substitute, like dialysis.

This often entails significant costs, financially and in terms of discomfort and adverse effects from treatment. After surgery, there's pain and disability. Medicines are likely to have side effects (cancer treatments in particular are tough, with the nausea and vomiting, hair loss, suppression of immunity, and malaise). It's about paying now for potential benefits down the road.

The alternative is palliative care, sometimes called comfort care. This refers to managing symptoms and treating the discomfort and disability, rather than focusing on curing the underlying condition. It's not about curing the cancer, but about tempering the associated symptoms. It's not about curing the liver failure, but about draining the ascites distending the abdomen. It's not about trying to resect the esophageal obstruction, but about placing a tube to allow the patient to swallow.

A good example of the emphasis is the common use of opiates for pain relief and sometimes for suppressing respiratory drive that causes such breathlessness and distress to people with end-stage COPD/emphysema or heart failure. The opiates depress respiration and are likely to hasten death, but the relief they bring justifies it.

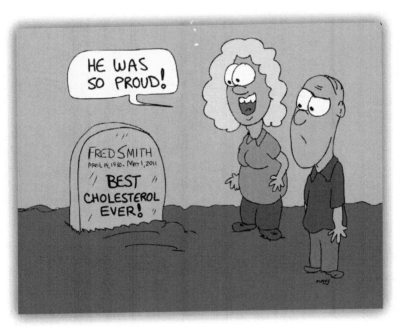

HOSPICE CARE

Speaking of palliative care, that's what hospice specializes in.

"Hospice" has the same linguistic root as "hospitality." Hospices were started by the Crusaders as one of their more compassionate, less pugilistic projects, to provide rest and shelter for the dying. The modern movement is attributed to Dame Cicely Saunders, a registered nurse turned medical social worker turned doctor who founded St. Christopher's Hospice in London, inspired by her experience of looking after a dying Polish refugee.

The focus of hospice is to make the end of life as meaningful and comfortable as possible, relieving symptoms and helping the patient remain as functional as possible. To quote the Hospice Foundation of America (www.hospicefoundation.org), it's a "special concept of care designed to provide comfort and support to patients and their families when a life-limiting illness no longer responds to cure-oriented treatments."

Hospice provides a "team of professionals and specially trained volunteers to address the medical, social, psychological and spiritual needs of the patient and family," writes Hank Dunn. Care is provided by a team that usually includes nurses, doctors, social workers, aides, counselors, therapists, spiritual advisors, and often lay volunteers to help with non-medical tasks. Hospice workers tend to really come into their own in the late stages to give emotional support and practical advice to caregivers. They are also accustomed to (and much better at) talking about death and dying, which so many other people are squeamish about, but which patients and caregivers need. Kübler-Ross pointed out that terminal patients often complain that nobody actually talks to them about dying.

In some ways, hospice is ahead of its time. It provides comprehensive care with a team of different types of providers, which is along the lines of this modern idea of medical homes, as mentioned in *Getting the Right Doctor*. It's a model we could all benefit from. It's a shame you have to be dying to take advantage of it.

Once enrolled in hospice, an individual care plan is drawn up. The hospice nurse has a special medical kit prescribed by the hospice or primary care doctor, allowing for administration of medicines for symptom control without the rigmarole of calling the doctor every time.

The most common location for people to get hospice care is at home, which is a great boon to those who want to die in familiar surroundings.

Recently, an old school friend of mine died after a long fight with esophageal and lung cancer. He'd turned to hospice when bone metastases kept spreading despite chemotherapy. He passed at home, in as good a way as can be, I'd say. His wife posted on Caring Bridge (a great site for keeping loved ones connected to someone experiencing a serious illness) that "The promise of hospice has been fulfilled—no—exceeded—in that both the patient and the family have been cared for in the most remarkable way . . . with pain minimal, our relief is palpable" and how the scene was "quite undramatic." Life went on in as usual a way as possible given the circumstances, until the end.

There are also hospice units in hospitals and nursing homes, as well as some freestanding facilities.

In his *The New Yorker* article, Gawande talks of going on a house call with a hospice nurse to visit a 72-year-old with congestive heart failure and pulmonary fibrosis. He talked to the patient and apparently pissed off the nurse by being somewhat crass and asking the patient why she'd chosen hospice care, to which the patient replied, "The lung doctor and the heart doctor told me they couldn't help me anymore."

Talking to the nurse afterwards, Gawande said he was confused by the treatment the patient was receiving. "Wasn't the goal of hospice to let nature take its course?"

"That's not the goal," remonstrated the nurse. "The difference between standard medical care and hospice is not the difference between treating and doing nothing," she explained; the difference is in the priorities of care.

Gawande is not alone in his idea. Three decades after hospice emerged as the standard of care for terminally ill patients, the end-of-life treatments that palliative medicine physicians provide are frequently called euthanasia, killing, and murder.

More than half of palliative medicine physicians say patients, family members, and even other health professionals have used those terms to describe care hospice recommended or implemented within the last five years, according to a nationwide survey of 663 palliative care doctors in the March 2012 *Journal of Palliative Medicine*.

Unfortunately, this tendency for people to consider hospice throwing in the towel, and the mistaken idea that doctors will ignore them and have no interest in treating them, deters a lot of people from getting on board sooner.

In truth, hospice provides a lot of care and attention, focused on comfort and function rather than a cure. It also helps the psychological/spiritual progression toward the end of life. "Families can get great healing when it's time to move away from an emphasis on efforts of curing the disease and moving toward reasonable and more meaningful goals," says Dunn. "To continue to fight for a cure when there is no reasonable hope for one may cut off the true growth and comfort that can come from going on this journey together with those we love."

Brody reports on a study that emphasizes this point. Dr. David Casarett, associate professor at the University of Pennsylvania's Perelman School of Medicine and director of Hospice and Palliative Care for the University of Pennsylvania Health System, and some colleagues interviewed family members of 100 patients two months after they died in hospice. All said there were aspects of hospice care they wished they'd learned of sooner. In particular, they mentioned the availability of the hospice team and visiting nurse twenty-four hours a day, the coordination of care services, and the spiritual and emotional support, which they had not realized they needed.

Patients getting there too late to really benefit from hospice seems to be a common theme. "The average length of stay in hospice is only 14 to 20 days," notes Angela Morrow, R.N., a former hospice guide, writing on About.com. But, "The work of the dying takes more time than the average length a patient is on hospice."

Rather than hospice being an abandonment of hope, a lot of people have hope rekindled when they learn that hospice combats the fear of pain and other kinds of suffering.

I remember a visit my aunt who had recurrent breast cancer that had not responded to treatment when she was in an assisted living facility in Buffalo. I joined her group of raucous, bantering seniors for breakfast as they ribbed Joe in his power wheelchair about his bad driving and repeatedly shuffled their walkers to the coffee urn for refills. Later, in a remarkably frank conversation about her future, she told me she wasn't afraid of dying. She, like so many others, was just afraid of suffering. Learning about what hospice provides can be a great comfort.

Because of this idea that calling in hospice is like calling in the Grim Reaper, Gawande reports on another study in which Aetna Insurance (with uncharacteristic wisdom) tried an experiment, letting a group with a life expectancy under one year continue their definitive treatments while simultaneously enrolled in hospice.

After two years, the terminally ill patients receiving this "concurrent care" showed a marked difference in their attitude toward hospice. Initially, only 26 percent accepted the idea of hospice, but by the end, there was an impressive 70 percent acceptance rate. But attitudes weren't the only things that changed. ER visits and ICU admissions dropped dramatically and—surely gratifying to Aetna—costs went down by 25 percent.

As a bit of an aside, in this and another Aetna study, the reduced utilizations by the patients seemed to be because they had someone available to give advice. "They had simply given patients someone experienced and knowledgeable to talk to about their daily needs. And somehow that was enough—just talking," notes Gawande.

Maybe there's a lesson here for more than just dying patients. One of my crazier friends once proposed that we need a toll booth kind of setup that people could drive through with their mystery symptoms, injuries, or whatever and ask a health professional, "Do I need to get seen for this?"

It sounded good until she suggested setting them up on Route 3, a traffic-choked main commuter road in Fredericksburg. But there's something to the idea of providing a mechanism for getting this sort of expert advice to people (I am aware that some insurance companies and websites have professionals available to advise). I'm sure it would greatly reduce the number of people showing up in the ER because they genuinely believe their hangnail could be life threatening.

Many also hold the not-unreasonable belief that people who change to palliative care/hospice die much sooner than those who plug along with definitive care.

Gawande admits he believed as much. Because patients forgo hospitalization and all the stuff that comes with it, like ventilators, dialysis, antibiotics, and artificial feeding, combined with common use of high-dose narcotics to combat pain, he "believed that hospice care hastens death."

Interestingly, this does not seem to be the case. Gawande reports on a study published in the *Journal of Pain and Symptom Management* in March 2007 that followed 4,493 terminal Medicare patients with one of five types of cancer or congestive heart failure, some in hospice and some not. The hospice patients did not die earlier. In fact, sometimes, "curiously, hospice care seemed to extend survival for some patients," he notes.

Another common misconception is that hospice is just for cancer patients. But Gazelle reports that nearly 40 percent of hospice patients suffer from end-stage cardiac disease, dementia, general debility, pulmonary disease, strokes, and other non-cancer problems.

Yet another impediment is that people sometimes think insurance doesn't cover hospice care. These days most insurance plans do pay for it, as long as patients meet the admission criterion of being expected to die within six months, which usually has to be certified by two doctors. Certification is for a limited time (six or nine months), after which the doctors have to re-certify, but this can be done repeatedly if the patient remains alive. Medicare has covered these services since the Medicare Hospice Benefit Act was passed in 1982.

The prejudice may be waning and the tide turning, according to Dr. Jonathan Bergman of the University of California, Los Angeles. He reports that in the last decade, hospice use has shown "a sharp increase."

Widespread dissemination of the taboo of "giving up" and of the need to soldier on with punishing treatments to the bitter end must change, asserts Morrow. "The population of seniors in the U.S. is expected to double in the next 30 years. That means more people will be living with chronic, life-limiting illness that need expert end-of-life care."

There is some opposition to hospice. Some religious organizations in particular get antsy about palliative care being a little too close to making God-like decisions. The Wisconsin Catholic Conference released a statement in July 2012 specifically criticizing a particular kind of detailed end-of-life instruction called POLST (which I'm getting to), and they "encourage all Catholics to avoid using all such documents, programs, and materials" as they consider them and living wills "real threats to the dignity of human life" that might be considered "an act of euthanasia."

A power of attorney is OK, the group says, but you are reminded to discuss your wishes and Catholic teachings with any healthcare proxy you appoint.

THE CONVERSATION ABOUT END-OF-LIFE WISHES

Hospice is an important topic for end-of-life care, but perhaps I'm getting a little ahead of myself. The "right" death begins earlier, with figuring out what you want and making sure those wishes are known by the appropriate people. It begins with "the conversation."

The Conversation Project (www.theconversationproject. org) is one of the more vigorous proponents of this talk. It encourages everyone, young or old, sick or not (accidents happen and life-threatening illness can strike at any age, as the organization warns), to have the conversation about end-of-life care wishes. It's mounting a campaign aimed at getting everyone together around the kitchen table to proactively and preemptively talk about what they would want.

When I think back to my own mother's death, it strikes me as a prime example of when this vital step is missing. It was a great illustration of how not to do things.

My mother was primarily a homemaker and devoted parent, but also a philanthropist on the boards and committees of various charitable organizations. She got breast cancer and underwent a mastectomy and radiation, and never got used to wearing a "falsey" to replace her missing breast. But everything seemed fixed and life got back to normal, with my sister working as a journalist for *The Guardian* in Manchester and me at medical school.

Our father was a psychiatrist, but one who relapsed to a rather infantile dependence on my mother, to whom he was devoted, as soon as he got home. She was happy to be mother to all three of us, such was her caretaker instinct.

Everyone always said, "it must be wonderful having a psychiatrist father who can analyze you." But my sister and I both understood that he would cast off his professional persona at home and resort to a neediness, presumably born of the rather disrupted childhood he had with parents, split between England and Germany. He would be his eccentric self and not the slightest bit psychoanalytical. I'd quip that he was the proof that mental illness is contagious.

At home one afternoon, about three years after her surgery, at the end of a year of complaining about a lack of energy and an inability to get going on a biography she wanted to write about my father's mother (a co-founder of the Summerhill School with A.S. Neill), my mother had a seizure.

To the med student I was then, it seemed surely indicative of a recurrence and spread of the cancer to her brain. I remember standing by as the local G.P., who came on a house call (as doctors in England did at that time) examined her, including the fundi of her eyes.

He uncomfortably nodded affirmation and said, "I think so" when I asked if he thought she had papilledema, a swelling of the optic disc indicative of raised intracranial pressure. In this circumstance, it was pretty much a *sine qua non* of brain metastases.

My father, despite being a doctor, just couldn't face the idea and was in complete denial. Reality set in when he officiously read the G.P.'s referral note to the admitting officer at the local hospital. Then there was this terrible atmosphere of grief and desperation, but still no open acknowledgment or discussion of the fact that my mother was dying and what her final wants and needs might be.

That difficult but all-important conversation was missing. Even though she was terminal, with no possibility for definitive care, there were management decisions to be made. They required some kind of open discussion, not just grief-stricken denial and despair.

A survey of terminal patients found their top priorities include avoiding suffering, being with family, experiencing the touch of others, being mentally aware, and not becoming a burden, notes Gawande.

But in her book, Bennett highlights a *JAMA* study finding that two-thirds of families don't recall ever having an end-of-life discussion. Studies show people are much more likely to have a "good death" (pain-free, at home if that's what they want, etc.) if they have a frank discussion of end-of-life strategy.

As noted, the medical profession's default position is to do everything. If the patient or decision-maker doesn't jump in and spell out what's wanted, the intervention train just keeps on a-rolling.

"Our healthcare system is really set up to cure the patient," notes JoAnne Reifsnyder, board president of the Hospice and Palliative Nurses Association. "If we can't cure, then folks sort of get confused about what do we do here? We have nothing in the toolbox."

If, as advocated by The Conversation Project, you've discussed with your loved ones what you want in the way of resuscitation, it'll probably be easier for important decisions to be made. If you haven't yet, but have some life-threatening illness, it's very important to talk now.

The conversation needs to be frank so everyone involved has a good handle on what's going on. It must cover the diagnosis and prognosis (the likely progression of the illness and the time line), as well as the pros and cons of any treatment options.

This brings us back to that old maxim I may have mentioned once or twice already: information is everything. Consult the most informed sources and your primary care doctor, whose knowledge and experience will be useful in figuring out how to best apply what your learn. A doctor specializing in your illness or affected part or system will be helpful too, particularly at a prestigious medical center or specializing hospital.

The problem is, some interventions are so new, and there's so much to keep up with these days, nobody knows it all. More importantly, every patient is different and no one can know exactly how someone will react to any given treatment.

Some guidance may be available in the form of a treatment's success rate statistics or an average five-year survival rate with a particular cancer on this particular drug, but that only provides probabilities, no certainties. If there's a 60 percent five-year survival rate for your particular cancer, there's of course no way of knowing whether you'll fall into the slim majority or not.

My aunt, who had stage IV breast cancer and metastases in her pleura—meaning fluid kept accumulating in the pleural space that compresses the lung and made her short of breath—was a good example.

To control the fluid accumulation, the oncologist offered chemotherapy in pill form, which sounded like a great idea. Except there's a good chance of some nasty side effects, worst of which is hand, foot, and mouth disease, involving multiple sores on the skin or lining of the mouth.

He also offered pleurodesis. This basically involves introducing an irritant into the pleural cavity to cause scarring that prevents the lungs from being compressed by fluid. Again, it sounds great, but some people experience severe pain. As a third option, a tube could be inserted to drain the fluid continuously, but there's a fair chance of infection.

It's very difficult to get accurate information about the probabilities of these complications. Would she experience a lot of pain from the pleurodesis or get hand, foot, and mouth disease? Exactly how effective would each method likely be in controlling the fluid? No one can really say; a decision like this involves a lot of guesswork.

Deciding what kinds of resuscitation or treatment to go for, or whether it's time to change from definitive to palliative care/ hospice is incredibly difficult. Not to mention, different family members may have passionately different opinions.

Also, if you have some setback that requires an intervention like CPR, a feeding tube, a ventilator, chemotherapy, or antibiotics to keep you alive, you must gamble on whether it's just a temporary problem after which you can regain a moderately comfortable and meaningful life or whether you're just prolonging your agony.

Obviously, a number of personal factors go into end-of-life care decisions. Everyone has to find their own way to the decision to abandon trying to beat the illness and switch to palliative care. The input of loved ones often plays a role, as do religious or philosophical beliefs.

As a Tibetan Buddhist, the Dalai Lama believes in reincarnation. When asked if he's afraid of dying, he answered with a shrug and a laugh and "Hah. Change of clothes."

Dare I say it, your insurance and financial status may influence things. Some newer interventions are insanely expensive, and if they're considered experimental, they may not be covered by insurance. It's part of our reality that some people simply can't afford the treatment needed to keep them alive.

WHEN TO HAVE THE TALK

The timing of the conversation is important. You need to have it before some radical intervention like a ventilator or a feeding tube becomes necessary.

Formulating a plan "often gets deferred until very late on—or doesn't happen at all," notes Morrow. Recognizing the benefits of an early start, other countries promote end-of-life planning.

"In Sweden, we have what we call a breakpoint conversation, a communication about the transition to end-of-life care," says Dr. Gunilla Lundquist, a palliative care specialist at Umea University in Sweden. It consists of a systematic series of talks that change the focus from prolonging life to providing comfort and physical, psychological, and spiritual support.

Gawande advises, "When the chemotherapy stops working, when we start needing oxygen at home, when we face high-risk surgery, when the liver failure keeps progressing, when we become unable to dress ourselves," these are the kinds of indicators that it's time to have the conversation.

But I take issue with him here. By these points, it's often too late to get the most out of palliative care, if that's going to be your choice.

It's important to have the conversation early on. Just keep in mind that circumstances may change. What seems right at one point may not seem right at a later date. Keep the conversation going and let it evolve as needed.

HAVING THE TALK WITH YOUR DOCTOR

Most people have "the conversation" with loved ones first. It's a good idea to broach the subject with your doctor, too, but it's also smart to be aware of some pitfalls. He may not always act like it, but remember, he's an ordinary mortal with emotional vulnerabilities when it comes to the nitty-gritty, and he may dissemble, minimize, avoid, etc. like anybody else.

Even if he's a specialist in the field, your doctor won't know everything. My friend Ernie with the prostate cancer went to a respected urologist, but had to find out for himself that you can get an MRI scan of the prostate to help locate the exact site of the cancer. The findings of his scan contributed to canceling the prostatectomy he was scheduled for.

Sometimes the doctor hasn't adequately filled you in, whether it's because there was insufficient time, you didn't ask the right questions (the doctor may not be good at seeing what information you lack, so be assertive and keep asking questions), or some other factor.

Sometimes the doctor is thinking in terms of probabilities. Sometimes he's holding out hope, knowing that everybody has the potential to react differently to any given treatment.

Just because someone's a doctor, just because he regularly deals with the sick and dying, that doesn't mean he's comfortable with death or talking about it.

I certainly remember instances of my discomfort and ineptitude dealing with dying patients and their families. The case of "Gum Drop" stands out in particular.

This was the name adopted by one of my patients who, with her husband ("Dr. C. Nile"), was one of a troop of clowns who dressed in giant shoes and red noses to do rounds at the local hospital on Saturdays to bolster the morale of patients and staff.

Gum Drop developed a host of obscure neurological symptoms, which turned out to be amyotrophic lateral sclerosis (ALS, or Lou Gehrig's Disease), which slowly paralyzes you until you basically die of asphyxiation.

Her husband was in for a blood pressure check and I asked him one of those open-ended questions we doctors are meant to ask so the patient can ramble on about any subject they think is important. "How are things at home?"

He looked glum and very un-clownlike and said in strained tones, "I don't like to think about the future."

In retrospect, this was surely a good opening to talk to him about how his wife was going to die and what could be done to help mitigate everyone's distress as much as possible. But no, I remember feeling a distinct discomfort and strong desire to move on. I started talking to him about his blood pressure medicine.

Because of such discomfort, and because nobody likes to be the bearer of bad news, many doctors tend to minimize or be unduly optimistic, especially when it comes to giving a prognosis.

Unfortunately, it takes very little encouragement from the doctor for a patient to be persuaded to try this or that treatment, to grasp at any straw.

Dr. Michael Grodin, director of medical ethics at Boston University School of Medicine and Public Health, says doctors should "provide support and be as realistic as possible." Being realistic means helping the patient rationally weigh the pros and cons of the potential courses of action.

Deciding how long a patient is going to survive is notoriously difficult, so sometimes the doctor either won't speculate or remains vague. But it's common for the patient or family to want to know, and the information can have a strong bearing on the choices at hand.

If a doctor underestimates how long a patient has to live, he's accused of destroying hope. "It's not [a doctor's] job to take away hope," says Michael Grodin.

So doctors tend to overestimate, corroborated by a study led by Harvard researcher Nicholas Christakis. Doctors of almost 500 terminally ill patients were asked to estimate how long they thought their patients would survive. Sixty-three percent over-estimated survival time by an average of 530 percent.

Interestingly, "The better the doctors knew their patients, the more likely they were to err." This presumably reflects the desire to not deliver horrible news, especially to someone with whom there's an established relationship.

Overestimating can deprive a person of the opportunity to work through important bucket-list items.

In her book, Brody talks about 65-year-old Arlene Wysong, a New York businesswoman diagnosed with incurable breast cancer. She opted for no chemo or other major interventions, saying "My goal from the beginning was to make sure I saw all the friends and family I wanted to see and spend quality time with them." Of particular importance, she wanted to work through "some serious issues that had caused a rift between her and her daughter."

She rewrote her will and made arrangements for her business. Sixteen months after she was diagnosed, she called in hospice and died peacefully at home with her family.

"Had Arlene's physician hemmed and hawed and failed to tell her just how serious her disease was" and overestimated her life expectancy, notes Brody, "she might have lived the remaining months with the fantasy that she might beat this cancer" and never have gotten to do important stuff like reconcile with her daughter.

And, I would add, she would likely have been subjected to the discomfort, disability, indignity, and expenses of hospital admissions, surgery, pain, nausea, weight loss, fatigue, sedation, mental confusion, diarrhea, hair loss, skin rashes, and the almost endless list of morbidities often associated with definitive treatments.

Gawande likens unrealistic expectations to a lottery. "We've created a multi-trillion dollar edifice for dispensing the medical equivalent of lottery tickets," but "have only the rudiments of a system to prepare patients for the near-certainty that those tickets will not win."

Adding to the doctor's discomfort are the unpredictable emotional reactions of patients. I know from experience if a patient is in the angry phase, he often apportions blame, possibly to the doctor for not having prevented the problem. Sometimes there's even every doctor's favorite topic of conversation: malpractice litigation. Other patients go into denial, not "hearing" what the doctor says, blowing it off as no big deal, or claiming there's a mistake and maybe they're going to see another (real) doctor.

At some point, the denial usually breaks down, and then the chance to talk further presents itself.

Doctors also tend to dance around the issue and never quite lay it on the line. They use jargon and talk about "a spot on the lung," "a shadow," "metastases," and the like, instead of using straightforward words like "cancer" that the patient is more likely to understand and appreciate the gravity of.

Sometimes the doctor doesn't have the conversation at all. If he's inhibited, you may need to take the lead and prod him along, giving him permission to talk about end-of-life care. One common tactic Gawande admits to is referring patients to specialists and letting them relay the bad news.

A piece on *The New York Times* website on November 16, 2011 by Paula Span reports the comments of Dr. Joan Teno, medical director of Home and Hospice Care of Rhode Island. She says the group has become accustomed to patients admitted with no clear understanding of their condition or prognosis. "The oncologist has told them, 'It's time to take a holiday from chemo,'" she says. "It's a way not to have a conversation he or she finds hard to do."

Hospice workers are particularly good at facilitating this kind of conversation and talking about death in general. They may give you a more realistic, reasonable take than your doctor. The catch-22 is you usually don't get to talk to these folks until you've already opted for palliative care.

People "who prepare for death by talking about it, sharing feelings, and being completely open leave behind survivors who are less plagued by guilt," notes Dr. Henry Rosberger, director of the Bereavement and Loss Center of New York.

I bet this would include your doctor. I bet doctors would feel less guilt about patient deaths if they had healthier end-of-life planning conversations with them.

ADVANCE DIRECTIVES

If the conversation results in an advance directive, it can prevent a lot of messes. In this document, also known as a living will, a person makes known his wants should he become ill and incapable of expressing them. It typically addresses what—if any— types of life-sustaining measures are desired. Often a person also appoints a healthcare proxy to make decisions if necessary.

Many people make an advance directive part of their regular will, with all their faculties still about them (hopefully). Everyone should do this, even the young. Accidents happen. Life-threatening illness can strike any time, and they don't dawdle to accommodate procrastinators.

You probably don't want to finish up like Terri Schiavo. She was 26 when she suffered massive anoxic brain damage from cardiac arrest. She was in a chronic vegetative state for 15 years while her husband petitioned the court multiple times to remove her feeding tube and let her die.

But her parents thought she might recover and that her existence was meaningful, so they opposed him. The whole thing became a national drama with President George W. Bush weighing in, siding with the pro-lifers by signing legislation aimed at keeping the feeding tube in.

It all could have been avoided if she'd had an advance directive, an irrefutable guide to her wishes that the court would've upheld.

Any treatment team needs to know specific stuff, like:

- Do you want CPR if your heart stops or you stop breathing? That's all the blowing and pumping to circulate oxygenated blood with the hope that things pick back up on their own. Or, there are drugs or defibrillation to kick the heart back on.

Reality isn't like the movies, however. If your heart stops due to a deteriorating disease process, the odds of it restarting are virtually nil. In his book, Dunn talks about how medical researchers reviewed 113 CPR studies over a thirty-three-year period and found the overall success rate was a dismal 15.2 percent.

Even if CPR does bring you back, it doesn't sound like people are any too enthusiastic about it. Dunn also cites a study of nursing home patients who were successfully resuscitated and discharged from the hospital; almost all refused any further CPR.

If you opt not to have CPR, your chart is usually labeled DNR for "do not resuscitate."

- Do you want intubation? That's when you put an endotracheal tube through the mouth into the trachea (airway) for long-term inflation of the lungs (otherwise, as in emergency CPR, you do mouth-to-mouth or use a bag and mask if they're available).

Having an endotracheal tube is very irritating, so usually the person has to be sedated, and they can't talk.

- Do you want to be put on a ventilator? This machine breathes for you by inflating your lungs. You have to be intubated, except in the old days of the "iron lung" for polio victims.

For long-term ventilation, a tracheostomy is usually performed. This entails making a hole in the front of your throat so a small tube can be inserted into the trachea without going through your mouth.

A ventilator can keep you alive for years, but you may never get strong enough to come off it. Then you or whoever's calling the shots may be faced with the decision of whether to "pull the plug" to stop the ventilator, likely resulting in death (though sometimes patients surprise everyone by continuing to breath on their own).

- Do you want to be fed artificially if you can't eat on your own? It typically involves a feeding tube down your nose or into your stomach or intestine through the abdominal wall. Sometimes, it's done by intravenous fluid with total parenteral nutrition.

It seems awful for someone to starve or thirst to death, and the idea tends to be unnerving for loved ones. But patients often give up eating and drinking in their final days; many cultures regard this as a sign of dying, not a cause.

Brody quotes palliative care specialist and psychiatrist Dr. Linda Ganzini of the Oregon Health and Science University School of Medicine, who says, "When a patient voluntarily refuses food, the result is nearly always a peaceful death."

The claim is that when you don't eat, the ketones your body produces by feeding off its reserves produces a euphoric, peaceful state of mind. Thought of like this, forgoing the feeding tube doesn't seem like such cruel and unusual punishment.

- Do you want medicines? You'll probably want analgesics or other medicines to relieve pain, nausea, anxiety, shortness of breath, and other uncomfortable symptoms. But when it comes to medicines that prolong life, sometimes it's a more knotty problem.

Pneumonia or a urinary tract infection are common terminal events when the body's defenses are overwhelmed. Generally, the patient just slips into unconsciousness and dies (pneumonia has been called "the old man's friend").

Prior to the 1950s, before antibiotics were so numerous and widely used, most deaths in North America were from infections. But with effective antibiotics for just about any infection, you now have to make a decision whether or not to treat. This can be difficult, requiring some guesswork as to whether the current predicament is a temporary problem from which you can bounce back.

- Do you want to be hospitalized? Dunn talks about having a "DNH" (do not hospitalize) order. In my experience, the majority of people want to die at home, but some are unnerved by the idea or worried they won't get adequate symptom control at home or in a nursing home.

If you opt to be admitted, be clear why and make relevant wishes known so as not get carried off by the definitive care onslaught if that's not what you want. Your advance directive should be in your hospital chart.

- One fairly new consideration, and a somewhat contentious issue, is what to do about people with an implanted pacemaker/defibrillator (ICD). These devices are programmed to provide an electrical shock to the heart to kick it back to life if it fails to work properly, which is what you normally want. But the problem is they almost won't let a person die.

In the past, doctors have refused to turn off ICDs, saying they'd cause the death of the patient. But patients and family members complain dying patients are effectively tortured. A report in the *Annals of Internal Medicine* quotes one family member of a dying patient saying of the defibrillator, "It went off 12 times one night." The claim is it's like being kicked by a mule.

It's since been established that a patient can refuse having an ICD kept on, as it's a right to refuse any treatment. The Heart Rhythm Society is reported in the May 2010 edition of amednews.com as having come up with guidelines that physicians "can deactivate defibrillators and pacemakers when terminally ill patients request it," which is very gracious of them.

So this is another issue you might express your wishes on.

In an effort to practice what we preach, my wife Paula and I both signed living wills and appointed healthcare proxies when we recently revised our wills.

Our lawyer provided us with a standard advance directive, which notes, "If at any time my attending physician determines I have a terminal condition where the application of life-prolonging procedures would serve only to artificially prolong the dying process" then I "direct that such procedures be withheld or withdrawn, and that I be permitted to die naturally." Just give me whatever is needed to alleviate pain and provide comfort.

This sounds impressive, but it doesn't spell out in detail exactly which measures we do and don't want. I'll get to discussing how this can be improved shortly.

With any kind of DNR, you're encouraged to file a copy somewhere safe, give one to your healthcare proxy and one to your lawyer, and to keep a copy in your wallet (or at least a note saying you have one). If you're debilitated or house-bound, consider wearing a special wrist band. Register your document with the U.S. Living Will Registry at www.uslivingwillregistry. com/howitworksind.shtm.

In some states, your advance directive has to be notarized. It's not a bad idea to do this wherever you live, just in case you run your car off the road or have a stroke in a state that mandates it.

Rescue squads require their own specific EMS DNR, sometimes called an out-of-hospital DNR, or OOH DNR. You need one of these if you don't want the squad to burst onto the scene in a frenzy of IV lines, endotrachial tubes, Ambu bags, and defibrillators to do their whole "load and go" routine with full CPR that puts any Indy 500 pit crew to shame. Remember, "do everything" is the default position, and that's what happens if you don't have the correct paperwork.

These special forms are unique in each state. Get an OOH DNR from your doctor and have several copies, as the squad will want one and the ER may want one if you're transported. This is the case even if you have a DNR on record in your hospital chart, because the ER is technically considered out-of-hospital, cautions The Eldercare Team, which provides detailed advice about this issue at www.eldercareteam.com/ public/606.cfm.

If you have an OOH DNR, display a copy somewhere prominent, like on the fridge, on your bedroom door, or above the head of the bed, so there's no delay finding it when time is of the essence to the EMTs itching to get started on CPR.

ALTERNATIVE DECISION MAKERS AND FUTILE CARE

The other common part of an advance directive is appointment of a power of attorney (POA), or a legal alternative decision maker who steps in should you become too incapacitated to call the shots.

If no POA has been named, the alternative decision maker is typically the next of kin, usually meaning a spouse, child, or parent. Sometimes, it's a court in contentious cases.

The guiding principal for an alternative decision maker is to do what they think the patient would want. However, there can be a lot of leeway here, and sometimes decisions aren't the most rational. "Families who are unprepared for what happens when death is imminent often panic and rush the patient to the hospital, where last ditch and usually futile attempts at resuscitation are made," says Brody.

Some families get into fights over what should be done. My observation is that it's usually some distant family member, someone who never normally has anything to do with the patient, who insists they want "everything done." This can cause real anguish within the family or medical staff when such efforts seem futile.

In such cases, it's often useful to turn to a more objective outside party. A doctor, hospice worker, religious leader, or even hospital ethics committee may prove helpful.

The most egregious example of a meddling family in my memory came with a total derelict of a patient I inherited on "big call" (when a doctor is assigned a patient who needs admitting but doesn't have a doctor). This guy would scratch together enough money to drink himself into a hepatic coma and get picked up by the rescue squad and deposited in the ER.

I'd get the call in the office. "Bucko's here again." I had to drop everything, abandon the patients in the office, and drive hell-for-leather to the hospital. I'd oversee the business of once again draining the fluid from his abdomen, supporting his circulation with IV fluid, administering a mass of vasopressor medicines, supporting his respiration with an endotracheal tube and ventilator, providing nutrition, administering antibiotics, providing skin and mouth care, arranging all the other stuff any comatose patient needs, and dragging this asshole back from the brink so he could go do it all over again.

After a few rounds it got old. Despite two meetings with the ethics committee, intended to impress upon the family—a crowd of almost equally disheveled kin who piled down *en masse* from West Virginia in their pickup—the futility of it all, they wouldn't listen.

They insisted it was God's will whether Bucko should live or die, and not for us to interfere. I always saw this perspective as a little contentious; is it God's will that all these interventions have been invented, or are we interfering by using them?

"Those that choose life-prolonging treatments for failing patients do so primarily out of an inability to let go and not out of moral necessity or medical appropriateness," says Dunn, citing two papers in the *Journal of the American Geriatrics Society* in 1993.

I think it's also born of unfamiliarity with what dying is really like. Formerly, people witnessed loved ones dying at home. Now, they die in the hospital, and most people don't observe this unsatisfactory, long, slow process of dwindling consciousness, coma, and gradually failing respiration that goes on for days. Instead, peoples' ideas of death are shaped more by the movies, with a loved one propping up on one elbow, saying something profound, then keeling over.

Dunn lays some blame at the feet of the treatment team also. "Sometimes it's easier to aggressively treat patients, perhaps even for years, than to help families confront the emotional and spiritual issues that are driving the treatment choices," he says.

Even when the patient is with it enough to call the shots, many get persuaded to go along with treatments they don't really want if their loved ones insist. In such cases, the doctors may be dealing with an emotional or unreasonable family pushing wrong decisions.

BETTER ADVANCE DIRECTIVES

Recognizing the need for detailed guidance for medical teams, various organizations have tried to improve on the process of having the conversation and converting it into an effective advance directive.

The Five Wishes booklet is probably the best known resource to help people provide detailed resuscitation directions. It was first put together in Florida in 1997 with assistance from the American Bar Association, the United Health Foundation, and a grant from the Robert Wood Johnson Foundation.

It specifically addresses:

- Who you want to make care decisions if you can't
- What kinds of medical treatments you do and don't want
- How comfortable you want to be
- How you want people to treat you
- What you want your loved ones to know

Five Wishes has been translated into many languages and released in Braille. Learn more at www.agingwithdignity.org/five-wishes.php.

In the 1990s, doctors in Oregon attempted to improve on the living will and help patients devise a systematic end-of-life plan. They implemented a program called Physician Order for Life-Sustaining Treatment (POLST).

It's much more specific and detailed than a regular advance directive. The person's wishes are noted in the medical record and signed as an order by the doctor. The forms are brightly colored to be easily found in the chart in a crisis, and the information is entered in an electronic database which first responders can access.

The POLST program encourages doctors to talk to their patients about terminal care early on—especially by the time they "would be surprised if the patient lived more than a year."

It has caught on and is being adopted by more and more states. A study in Lacrosse, Wisconsin showed 85 percent of nursing home residents had a POLST, and consequently "few nursing home residents are transferred to the hospital," notes the *Managing Healthcare Costs* blog.

As a testament to efficacy, people with POLSTs indicating only comfort care were 59 percent less likely to receive unwanted life-sustaining treatments than people with conventional DNRs, according to a report in the *Journal of the American Geriatrics Society*. The hope would be that *no one* with a DNR would be resuscitated, but it happens, such is the enthusiasm for keeping people alive.

The report also found that people with a POLST who also opted to carry on with definitive treatment got as good treatment as someone without a DNR. This contradicts the notion that after you sign any kind of advance directive you're just tucked up in bed and left to gently fester and fade away.

To find much more detailed advice than I can provide, I recommend two books in particular: Hank Dunn's *Hard Choices for Loving People*, which focuses on emotional/personal/spiritual issues, and Brody's comprehensive *Guide to the Great Beyond*, which includes a section on terminal care of children and examines the idea of your legacy.

Also, check out *Understanding Your Living Will: What You Need to Know Before a Medical Emergency* by Dr. Ferdinando L. Mirarchi, chairman of emergency medicine at Hamot Medical Center in Erie, Pennsylvania. It provides lots of information on the specifics of your advance directive and discusses in detail how to make these kinds of tough decisions about exactly what you want in the way of resuscitation.

The Affordable Care Act tried to facilitate meaningful end-of-life counseling from doctors by providing special payments for them. This recognized that counseling takes time, and, as mentioned previously, that "cognitive" services are not nearly as well reimbursed as procedures.

Unfortunately, certain blowhard politicians cast these as "death panels," so what would have improved things became a political football and the funding got stripped from the bill. The Liverpool Care Plan, a comprehensive end-of-life palliative care plan in Britain, fell foul of the same kind of critics.

PREPARING FOR DEATH

As noted, most people aren't too familiar with the process of dying, but knowing what to expect can be a great help to both patient and caregiver. Certain emotional and practical preparations make it easier.

A dying person is more ready to go after taking care of their last to-do list. This isn't quite the same as a "bucket list," which is a longer term consideration of things someone always wanted to do.

The final to-do list generally includes things like seeing and saying goodbye to particular people (though many people getting close to death tend to withdraw socially), making peace with anyone with whom there's been conflict, getting business or legal affairs sorted out, making sure papers/files are findable to help out the executor, and even just organizing things around the house. Brody talks of one man who labeled the fuse boxes and cabinet draws for his wife before he died.

There are less tangible things to think about, like a legacy. In his book *Healthy Aging*, Andrew Weil talks about writing an "ethical will." This "has to do with non-material gifts: the values and life lessons you wish to leave to others." This is a practice strongly associated with Jewish tradition from thousands of years ago, he notes, but one that's making a strong comeback.

Understanding the dying process really helps the caretaker in particular. A frank conversation with a doctor or hospice worker is useful in this regard. Expecting the person to socially withdraw, to lose interest in eating and drinking, to sleep a lot, to be disorientated or even seeing visions, to gradually become less responsive, and to make gurgling noises as secretions gather (callously referred to as "the death rattle" by irreverent young doctors) can make it easier to bear witness to.

Saying goodbye and giving the person permission to die are very emotive but important tasks for the caregiver. Then, it's good to know what to do with the body and what arrangements have to be made. When my father died, I was clueless, but luckily I was dating a woman whose father had recently passed and who was a bit of take-charge feminist anyway, so she was wonderfully helpful.

A funeral or memorial service is a good way to focus the grief, but it doesn't have to be all doom and gloom. Just look at Irish wakes. My sister and mother's funerals were sad affairs for my father, but I remember lots of distant relatives coming to the house and it being something of a reunion party.

Some say it's such a shame the dead person doesn't get to hear all the nice things people say about them and suggest that funerals should be held before death. But maybe friends and relatives wouldn't be so gushing if the "the deceased" wasn't?

For further help, Brody's book has a lot of practical advice, as does Hospicenet.org at www.hospicenet.org/html/preparing_for-pr.html.

CARETAKER BURNOUT

With all this talk of end-of-life care, I'd be remiss not to mention a common affliction arising in the loved ones of the dying: caretaker burnout.

"The best way to take care of your loved one is pay attention to your own health," says writer and speaker Dr. Beth Erickson on Strengthforcaring.com. "It serves no one if you are worn to a frazzle because of your devotion."

Caretaking is an honorable but exhausting business that can completely eclipse the caretaker's normal life. Often, it's someone with no relevant training. Burnout is especially likely to strike if you're dealing with a person needing attention night and day, interrupting your sleep, and making you anxious. It's quite common in those caring for someone with dementia, between witnessing the devastation and having to constantly be on guard against the loved one wandering off or burning down the house; with something like Alzheimer's, this can go on for years. It's liable to break down even the strongest person.

Typical signs of burnout include mood swings between anger, sadness, hopelessness, and irritability; sleeping badly; not eating enough or sometimes eating too much; social withdrawal; and pretty much any other stress-related symptom.

Caretakers face guilt about leaving loved one. There's the fear of them dying while away (which sometimes seems to happen by intent, as I'll get to soon) and the mistaken notion that it's unacceptable to do something pleasurable while your loved one is dying. These sort of concerns prevent people from taking proper breaks from their caretaking duties.

The most basic prevention advice is all that healthy living stuff, like eating right, getting enough sleep (most people need seven to eight hours), and exercising for at least twenty minutes three times per week, doing something like brisk walking that gets you a little out of breath.

You may object that you don't have time for these remedies, but "Finding time for oneself is the most frequently reported unmet need of family caregivers," says a Caregiving in America report from 2006.

Social connections have never been more important. You need someone to talk to, to unload on. This can mean friends or family, and it's preferable to meet in person, but talking by phone is second best. Also, various websites connect people dealing with the same stresses. The Johnson and Johnson site www.strength-forcaring.com and www.cancercare.org are two examples.

Hospice can arrange for someone to step in to provide a break. The Agency on Aging (www.n4a.org) also provides help and advice. Congregants at your church or other religious institution are often happy to help out. Don't be afraid to delegate, either. People will ask if there's anything they can do; write down a list and refer to it when people inquire.

Sometimes the stress pushes people into full-blown anxiety or depression, which may need medical treatment. Caregivers are often so consumed by it that they don't recognize problems in themselves. Don't be dismissive of the concerns of others, even if you think it's just because they don't understand what you're dealing with.

If you're the busy, competent one in the family, there's a high risk most of the caretaking responsibilities will get dumped on you if some relative needs tending to. The only wise thing one particularly obnoxious attending surgeon told us when I was a medical student was, "If you want to get something done, give it to someone who's busy."

You shouldn't have to do all the other chores, especially if you're the one always physically present. Find the strength to be assertive. If your time's spent attending to a dying loved one, it's reasonable to not have to arrange the kids' carpool, the office outing, and the church yard sale. Learn to say no.

Finally, be aware that your whole life has been disrupted and put on hold to do this honorable and loving task. When your loved one dies, life reverts to normal, except for the large hole left by the sudden absence, of course. Suddenly your days are completely different. Prepare mentally for when this happens. Think about how it will be afterward and plan for returning to daily life, and maybe even for a getaway first.

DECIDING TO DIE

My impression, supported by others, is that people have some control over when they die.

Brody tells of a friend who sat at her companion's hospital hospice bed for weeks. "But the very day the hospice nurse encouraged her to take a break was the day he died." She speculates that dying people don't want their loved ones to witness the event, "which is anything but glamorous."

"It seems that some dying people actually choose the moment of their departure to coincide with their loved one's leaving the room," says hospice nurse Susan R. Dolan.

I've seen many instances of someone who is dying apparently holding on until a particular friend or relative comes to visit. Then they let go and die shortly after. And sometimes it seems loved ones need to give the patient permission to die.

Conversely, I had an uncle diagnosed with late-stage cancer (he apparently kept quiet about any symptoms) who was told by the oncologist he would live for a few months. He died two days later. My sense of it was he didn't want to be a bother and somehow sped the process along.

The physiology of how you hasten your death isn't understood, though it is recognized that there can be some degree of conscious control over some supposedly unconscious functions, like heart or metabolic rate. It's a trick yogis seem to have learned.

ASSISTED SUICIDE

Deciding to die can be less subtle, as sometimes the right death means an accelerated death.

This may sound radical, and it's ethically controversial, but physician-assisted suicide (PAS) or physician-assisted death (as some prefer) can be merciful for suffering patients—and their loved ones—especially when intractable pain is involved. As of this writing, PAS is permitted in four states.

Oregon was the first state to allow it, enacting the Death with Dignity Act in October 1997. Washington and Vermont followed suit, and PAS in Montana is not prosecuted.

To qualify, strict criteria must be met. In Oregon, the patient has to be mentally competent and the doctor needs to be as certain as possible depression isn't prompting the desire to die. Also, two doctors must certify that the patient's illness will kill him within six months. The patient has to make a written request, confirmed by two witnesses, and then a second request at least fifteen days after the first.

If the patient hasn't died by then, the doctor prescribes a lethal dose of a barbiturate like secobarbital, which induces sleep and suppresses respiration, causing death in an average of just over half an hour.

The PAS initiative has been supported by various organizations, like Compassion and Choices. It provides information for anyone considering such an option at www.compassionand-choices.org. As with the abortion debate, anything where lives are deliberately ended raises moral and religious objections, and any doctor or pharmacist with objections doesn't have to participate.

Multiple challenges to these laws have been made. In Oregon, there have been numerous appeals through the courts, a challenge in the Supreme Court by the Bush administration, and an attempt by then-Attorney General John Ashcroft to suspend the licenses of doctors prescribing for PAS. A statewide ballot defeated a measure trying to overturn the Death with Dignity Act, and to date the law has been upheld.

Opponents in Oregon worried people would pour into the states where PAS is available to bump themselves off. Legislators tried to avoid this by making residency a requirement, though they didn't specify any required length of residency time.

There hasn't been any stampede of people wanting to end it all. According to Brody, "In Oregon, only 1 percent of patients in terminal stages of illness have asked for a lethal prescription that could hasten their death, and only 0.1 percent have received approval or followed through."

Only 255 lethal prescriptions were written in the first three years of legal PAS in Washington, where there are 50,000 deaths per year. One participating clinic, the Seattle Cancer Care Alliance, reported 40 percent of its patients didn't use the prescription.

Dr. Elizabeth Trice Loggers, medical director of palliative care at this clinic, says even unused prescriptions are liberating, offering the knowledge that a means of escape is available. "Just having the option, the choice, to choose one's fate has actually increased the willingness to talk to one's family and doctor about other choices. That includes palliative care, like hospice, and even life-extending therapies they may not have wanted to try before," she explains, adding, "Families have expressed gratitude for the program."

Some think PAS hasn't gone far enough, and that people should be able to get help ending their suffering from people other than doctors.

This includes Lawrence Egbert, M.D., an 83-year-old retired anesthesiologist and medical director of Final Exit Network (FEN). He's been dubbed "The New Dr. Death," inheriting the mantle from Dr. Jack Kevorkian. When Egbert came to speak at our local Unitarian Fellowship (he is a Unitarian Minister as well), I thought the elderly, soft spoken, slightly overwhelmed seeming man with a white goatee looked more like Colonel Sanders than Dr. Death.

He's also not as flamboyant and in-your-face as Kevorkian, who drove around the country in his VW minibus with his suicide machine and made a video tape in 1998 of himself administering a lethal injection to a 53-year-old man with ALS that was shown on *60 Minutes* (immediately before *Touched by an Angel*, incidentally).

FEN members act as "exit guides" who advise but don't physically assist or supply equipment. Not that this has stopped the multiple attempts in different states to prosecute Egbert and his associates.

Their favored method is asphyxiation with a helium-filled plastic hood. Given that breathing helium makes you talk like a munchkin, I imagine this detracts from the gravitas of someone's final words.

As is often the case, the U.S. has a more conservative stance than many other countries. The Netherlands, renowned for its social liberalism, goes a step further, allowing euthanasia (it became the first country to legalize it in 2002). With euthanasia, the doctor administers the fatal dose, while PAS requires patients to take it for themselves in pill form. That poses a problem if the patient is too debilitated or can't swallow.

Euthanasia typically involves an injected barbiturate like thiopentone. This is followed by a paralyzing agent like pancuronium, a chemical pharmacologically related to the South American arrow poison curare, which paralyzes the muscles, including those of respiration, causing asphyxiation. Scary as it sounds, this is the exact same combo used to anesthetize, but then the patient is on a ventilator so he doesn't die.

I can tell you from my stint in anesthetics in Britain, anesthetizing means holding people in a precarious balance between life and death, often for hours while the surgeon hacks away. The anesthetist's maxim is "95 percent of the time bored to death, 5 percent of the time scared to death."

This medicine combo is also used in executions by lethal injection, along with potassium chloride to stop the heart, a complication ideally avoided in anesthetized patients.

There are a lot more mercy killings in the liberal Netherlands. Reportedly there are some 2,300 to 3,100 per year in a population of about seventeen million. Opponents of the practice claim the figure is much higher because many cases aren't registered.

An even more radical service called "Life End" (*Levenseinde*) has been started in The Netherlands by The Dutch Association for a Voluntary End to Life. This is a team that travels around the country performing euthanasia on the patients of doctors who refuse to be involved (shades of Kevorkian).

Although euthanasia is not legal in the U.S., the reality is a lot of people in their terminal phase are helped along by large doses of opiate pain medicines, which like barbiturates suppress the respiratory system and lead to respiratory arrest. Withholding fluids is another maneuver that hastens death.

ORGAN DONATION

Not to sound too cliché, but death can have more meaning if it offers life to someone else. Just because a person dies, that doesn't mean all their organs and tissues are beyond use. It's becoming increasingly feasible to transplant them.

You may have heard about heart, kidney, liver, lung, and cornea transplants. But now it's possible to transplant a pancreas, intestine, connective tissue, skin, bone, marrow, and more, so think of yourself as a repository of spare parts for a lucky recipient.

The bad news is there's a woeful lack of organs available. The Health Resources And Service Administration notes that in 2013, there were 121,272 people waiting for transplants, but only 14,257 donors. Estimates vary, but somewhere between 5,000 and 6,000 people die each year for lack of an available organ.

Despite this, "Organs ... are recovered from less than 50 percent of actual potential donors, resulting in the loss of thousands of life-saving transplants," notes Robert Metzger, M.D., president-elect of the United Network for Organ Sharing.

Various suggestions have been offered for increasing donor rates. The LifeSharers (www.lifesharers.org) organization signs up willing donors and gives them preferred access should they ever need an organ, as a sort of *quid pro quo*.

Some have suggested paying for donated organs/tissues, and organs are sold on black markets in some parts of the world. Nancy Scheper-Hughes, writing in *The New Internationalist*, condemns this as "the new cannibalism."

As most people are aware, you can indicate on your driver's license if you're willing to be a donor. In the U.S., this is an opt-in arrangement, and state donor rates average 45 percent (they're as low as 5 percent in Vermont). In many European countries, where you instead have to opt out, more than 90 percent of citizens are donors, reports Brody.

Even if you're young and healthy and haven't yet given much thought to dying or passing on your parts, you could always be killed in a car crash tomorrow, so I urge you to sign up to be an organ donor today.

Fortunately, as I discuss in *Getting the Right Future*, there are some advances like 3D printers that may alleviate the organ shortage.

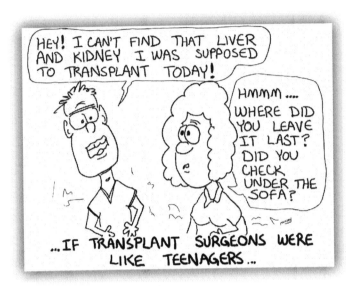

... IF TRANSPLANT SURGEONS WERE LIKE TEENAGERS ...

THE FINANCIAL COST OF TERMINAL CARE

Poorly managed end-of-life care doesn't only have major emotional costs; it often precipitates horrendous bills for little to no benefit. It is a significant part of the runaway cost of the healthcare that's such a drag on the U.S. economy.

"The soaring cost of healthcare is the greatest threat to the country's long-term solvency," claims Gawande, and "the terminally ill account for a lot of it."

In *The Cost of Hope*, Bennett asks why her husband ran up bills of $43,711 for one admission, $33,382 for another (after the doctors said he only needed comfort care) and $14,022 for a third in the last three days of his life.

Over the course of his disease, Bennett's husband had seventy-six CAT scans (with a price tag of $618,616) and multiple other interventions and tests ordered in an unthinking way without consideration for, or discussion of, the big picture.

In his article "Bitter Pill," Steven Brill tells the story of a man named Steven D. who was diagnosed with lung cancer in January 2011 who "kept saying he wanted every last minute he could get, no matter what." His wife Alice knew they were only buying time, but "How much is time really worth?" she asked. She made about $40,000 per year and had to think about how all the debt they were incurring would leave her and her daughter.

By the time Steven D. died at his home the following November, he had lived an additional eleven months, and his wife Alice had collected bills totaling $902,452.

Also illustrative of how much end-of-life care costs is the fact that 25 percent of Medicare spending is for the 5 percent of patients in their final year of life. Most of that money goes for care during the last couple of months—care which is often of little or no real benefit. Each year, Medicare spends more than the annual budget for Homeland Security or the Department of Education (more than $50 billion per year) on patients' last two months of life, reports *60 Minutes.*

This equates to using "about a third of our overall health-care resources in the last year of life," notes a report in *Reuters Health*, quoting Bergman. This "represents a huge avenue for improvement," he points out.

"Improvement" is a nice way of saying "savings," but I suppose talking about trying to gain huge savings by reducing or withholding treatments from dying patients may seem a little politically incorrect to some.

Some of the newer treatments, which everyone wants, of course, are insanely expensive. The new wonder drug Folotyn for a form of lymphoma costs $30,000 per month. Incidentally—because I just can't help myself—it received accelerated approval from the FDA even though "There's been no proof of even life extension," notes Jeff Levin-Scherz from the Harvard School of Public Health. Soliris, made by Alexion Pharmaceuticals, treats the rare blood disease paroxysmal nocturnal hemoglobinuria and a kidney disorder called atypical hemolytic-uremic syndrome. According to *Forbes*, it's the most expensive drug in the world, with an annual price tag of $440,000 for one patient.

The more common stuff, like ICU care, MRI and CT scans, and surgery, may cost less, but they're still expensive and wrack up enormous spending in a short time. These are all generally cure-oriented interventions, and ordering them mindlessly without regard for cost or big-picture benefits is a large part of why we spend so much at the end of peoples' lives.

These expenses show no sign of abating, though Bergman holds out hope as more people opt for hospice. Patients receiving hospice care typically forgo life-saving or potentially curative but expensive treatments like chemotherapy.

"Instead they receive treatment of their symptoms, as well as assistance with their spiritual and social needs," which is likely to result in the unlikely combination of better care for less money. It is "bringing these costs down while improving patient care," Bergman says.

Urging people to choose palliative rather than definitive care to save money may seem a little controversial, but as noted earlier, many people wish they'd opted for palliative care sooner once they get there and come to understand its many benefits.

We have limited resources, and when you spend masses of money on one thing, you tend to de-fund another. You're robbing Peter to pay Paul. So there is less money for less sexy but eminently more sensible prevention programs like immunizations, education programs to reduce obesity or stop smoking, better training for more primary care doctors, and the like (and the $15 billion allocated for the ACA's Prevention and Public Health Fund already had $6.5 billion chopped out by Congress' Deficit Reduction Package).

Sometimes, sensible allocation has to be enforced, as when everyone wants the newest and most expensive option available. Unless we suddenly become willing to go the unpopular route of paying ever-increasing insurance premiums or higher taxes for government programs, everyone can't have the best—or the costliest—of everything.

Other countries have panels of experts to help make these difficult decisions about where money is best allocated. But as I've said, this has been shot down by blowhard politicians and labeled with inflammatory names like "death panels" and "rationing" whenever anyone introduces such an idea in the U.S.

MEDICAL MARIJUANA

It's debatable whether this topic belongs in this chapter or if it might be better suited to the earlier conversation on complementary and alternative treatments, but I'll let you worry about that, I guess. It's certainly relevant to symptom control at the end of life.

Marijuana is dried flowers and subtending leaves of the cannabis plant. It contains 483 compounds, eighty-four of which are cannabinoids, the most significant of which is tetrahydrocannabinol (THC), its principal psychoactive compound. These substances are also in the resin the plant produces, which is made into hashish.

These compounds get you high, but they also have a lot of potential medical uses. Marijuana's been tried for an enormous array of physical and psychological illness, but is mainly used for terminal illnesses like HIV and cancer to treat pain and nausea (especially from chemo). But other well-known uses include for seizures and muscle spasms, and the refined derivative canasol is used for glaucoma.

The medicinal effects have been known for eons. Cannabis is one of the fifty "fundamental herbs" of traditional Chinese medicine. There are recipes for its use in Egyptian papyri, including one for cannabis suppositories for the relief of hemorrhoids. The ancient Greeks used it as a veterinary remedy and it's been used in India medicinally and for worship.

When I drove "the Hippie Trail" to India, I met many of those traveling ascetics, the Sadhus, who, like Rastafarians, smoke ganja as part of their religious practice. They were impressively devout, if judged by how many chillums they smoked in the course of their devotions.

There's a lot of skepticism about how useful medicine marijuana is, but a composite analysis of thirty-eight randomized controlled trials published in *The Clinical Journal of Pain* in February 2013 noted 71 percent demonstrated statistically significant pain relief. A report in the *British Journal of Clinical Pharmacology* on cannabinoids for the treatment of non-cancer pain concluded, "Overall, there is evidence that cannabinoids are safe and modestly effective in neuropathic pain with preliminary evidence of efficacy in fibromyalgia and rheumatoid arthritis."

The website ProCon.org reports on a combination of 105 human and animal studies of cannabis and cannabis extracts for treating a variety of conditions. It concludes that 39.05 percent were pro, 31.43 percent were con, and the rest were "not clearly pro or con."

As with any medicine, people worry about safety. Its millennia of use, the general lack of adverse effects (unless you consider getting stoned an adverse effect—but the pharmaceutical industry is working hard to eliminate that wicked euphoriant effect), and no known death from overdose are all encouraging.

The adverse effect people worry about most is whether marijuana has any long-term detrimental effect on brain function, and particularly motivation. Stoners have been known to display that "motivational inertia" people talk about.

There is also some concern that cannabis affects brain structure, and fMRI scans show some consistent alterations in brain function. However, "The relation of these changes to cognitive functioning is less clear." There's fairly good evidence it messes with your hippocampus and interferes with remembering things, notes the National Institute on Drug Abuse of the National Institute of Health (NIH).

There are accusations that marijuana is addictive, though I hasten to point out that this isn't a particularly pressing concern for terminal patients. Not to mention there's a widespread acceptance of opiate pain medications, with which the addiction concern is much more founded.

Subtle withdrawal symptoms have been observed following regular use, with some similarities to nicotine withdrawal, including irritability, sleeping difficulties, cravings, anxiety, and increased aggression on psychological tests.

Addiction is defined as compulsive, out-of-control use continuing in the face of detrimental effects and a tendency for use to escalate. The National Institute on Drug Abuse claims there is a 9 percent addiction rate, and 18 percent of those in treatment for addiction say cannabis is their primary drug.

But there are plenty of people using it in whom "use doesn't escalate over time," notes J. Wesley Boyd, M.D., Ph.D., Harvard Medical School faculty member and attending psychiatrist at Cambridge Health Alliance, writing in the November 2013 *Psychology Today*. "They can enjoy its effects without endangering some major element of their lives," he says. Then there are people "in the realm between the casual user and the full-on addict that I label 'almost addicted,'" he adds, but cautions that just because the majority don't get addicted, that doesn't mean it isn't potentially addictive.

Another question is whether marijuana is a "gateway drug." A study of over 300 pairs of fraternal and identical twins found the twin who'd used marijuana before the age of 17 had elevated rates of other drug use and drug problems later on, notes the NIH. It raises the question, though, whether marijuana is the cause, or whether a personality drawn to marijuana is more likely drawn to other experimentation. One facetious response on the website says marijuana is a dangerous gateway drug "that can lead to more serious addictions like Guitar Hero and Doritos and working retail until you are 50."

Some research has suggested a negative effect of THC on the function of various immune cells, but "no studies to date connect marijuana's suspected immune system suppression with greater incidence of infections or immune disorders in humans," notes the site.

There is also concern that, like cigarettes, inhaling marijuana smoke may be harmful to the lungs. But in 2012, an NIH-funded study published in the *Journal of the American Medical Association* examining marijuana's effects on the lungs concluded that smoking the equivalent of one joint per day for seven years "was not associated with adverse effects on pulmonary function."

There was however a paper in the *International Journal of Cardiology* in 2006 suggesting marijuana may cause a variety of heart problems, including being a "more common cause of myocardial infarction than is generally recognized."

Lester Grinspoon, associate professor emeritus of psychiatry at Harvard Medical School, is obviously undaunted. "When cannabis regains its place in the U.S. pharmacopoeia," a status it lost after passage of the Marijuana Tax Act of 1937 (which was really directed at hemp production), "it will be seen as one of the safest drugs in that compendium."

Its classification as a schedule I narcotic has inhibited the drug's medical use. Regarding marijuana as some wicked narcotic is a very recent view. The change in perception is mostly attributable to misinformation bandied about by Harry J. Anslinger, the first commissioner of the Federal Bureau of Narcotics, who launched a nationwide media campaign with the infamous *Reefer Madness* movie, claiming, "Smoke marihuana cigarettes for a month and what was once your brain will be nothing but a storehouse of horrid specters. Hashish makes a murderer who kills for the love of killing out of the mildest mannered man who ever laughed at the idea that any habit could ever get him."

And I thought it just mellowed you out.

Still, the American Society of Addiction Medicine has just changed its stance to acknowledge that research in the last few decades has pointed to potential therapeutic uses. This comes after long maintaining there was no such thing as medical marijuana because the plant parts in question fail to meet the standard requirements for approved medicines.

Other organizations are slowly coming around to similar acknowledgments. As of this writing, the FDA hasn't approved marijuana as safe and effective for any use. "The agency has, however, approved one drug containing a synthetic version of a substance that is present in the marijuana plant and one other drug containing a synthetic substance that acts similarly to compounds from marijuana but is not present in marijuana," says the website.

Twenty-three states and the District of Columbia allow use for medicinal purposes as of this writing.

A recent visit from Paula's friend Rick, who has pancreatic cancer and a pharmacy container of medical marijuana, makes me think there may not be a sea of separation between medication and recreation.

He describes his visit to the dispensary, where as a first-time customer, he chose a "welcome to our dispensary" present of a joint or cannabis cookie. He chose his medicine from a formulary of distinctly non-medicinal names like "Northern Lights," "Cinderella 99," "Dutch Haze," and "Purple Kush."

In November 2009, those stoners at the AMA adopted a new policy urging the Federal government to review the status of marijuana as a schedule I narcotic in an effort to make it easier to perform research on cannabis. It was careful to specify that this was not an endorsement, though.

The first step in getting a prescription for medical cannabis is living in a state where it's legal, though some states accept out-of-state cards.

For information on what's covered and about the process of getting a prescription, go to www.wikihow.com/Get-Medical-Marijuana. ProCon.org explains different state regulations at http://medicalmarijuana.procon.org.

Usually, your doctor has to sign a statement confirming your diagnosis and his recommendation for marijuana. You then apply to the state for your card, pay the fee, and head for the dispensary, which, as noted, is more like an Amsterdam coffee shop than a CVS or Walgreen's.

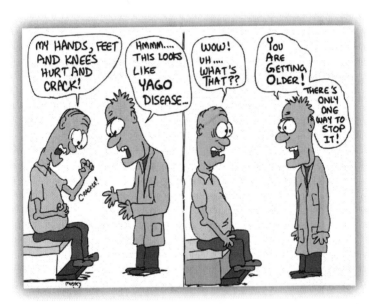

A LAST THOUGHT

The abhorrence of death that pervades the medical profession also involves the population as a whole. We spend massive amounts of money to continue to populate this overcrowded planet.

We need a change of attitude. We need to once again accept this inevitability with philosophical composure rather than freaked-out rejection.

We need an updated *Ars moriendi.*

CHAPTER 7

GETTING THE RIGHT FUTURE

———◆———

SCIENCE FICTION BECOMES NONFICTION

SURGERY PERFORMED BY ROBOTS, SOMETIMES operated thousands of miles away from the patient; brain cell scanners that can tell if you're lying; smartphone apps to check yourself for STDs; injectable "minibots" nearly as thin as a human hair that traverse your blood vessels; contact lenses that change color or tattoos that fluoresce to indicate blood sugar problems; replacing faulty inherited genes with healthy ones; contraception from an implanted microchip you can turn on and off with a scanner.

It's the stuff of science fiction, only it's not fiction. It's here already and transforming healthcare. The claim is that rapidly evolving technology will alter the business of medicine as much in the next fifty years as it did in the last 500.

Some of the information in this section isn't as immediately applicable or actionable as the information in other sections, and many innovations are prohibitively expensive. But this will change.

Doctors can't keep up with everything that comes along. That's why it's to your benefit to know what's currently emerging and coming down the pipeline.

EVER-EVOLVING HEALTHCARE

Until about 500 years ago, medicine was an empirical business pervaded by unscientific ideas like illness being caused by miasmas or out-of-balance humors. Treatments often had no rational basis, and not infrequently, they did more harm than good (e.g., bleeding and purging patients already in circulatory collapse, treating syphilis with mercury, treating asthma with cigarettes, using radium as a tonic, plombage for treating TB, and trepanning). The gullible public was persuaded to accept these often horrific treatments by the omniscient self-confidence of the doctors.

Dare I say it, that still happens today.

Gradually, the scientific method took over with treatments based on rational observation and deduction. It became the religion of evidence-based medicine, epitomized by dogmatic reliance on clinical trials. With advances in information technology especially, progress seems on an exponential trajectory, though medicine has a well-founded reputation for conservatism and being slow to embrace innovation.

It's sometimes tempting to think we must have learned most of what there is to know by now (a hubristic notion expressed from time to time throughout the evolution of medicine with major advances like asepsis, anesthesia, and antibiotics). But we're still in diagnose-and-treat mode, rather than having achieved the ultimate in healthcare: predict and prevent. Preventive care, for a variety of reasons, has not been a particularly prominent feature of medicine in the U.S.

As a disclaimer, there's an enormous amount of innovation taking place, and it's hard to predict what will hit the jackpot. I picked out things I think are the most important, but can only give you my take, which is a bit of a snapshot of this moving target.

GENOMICS

Arguably, the field yielding the most revolutionary changes recently—and the one best suited to enhancing our ability to predict and prevent illness—is genomics. This is the branch of molecular biology concerned with the structure, function, evolution, and mapping of all human genetic material.

On June 26, 2000, there was much excitement and fanfare at a White House reception. Bill Clinton was in an expansive mood. Tony Blair was participating from London via video link. Arch rivals J. Craig Venter from Celera Corporation and Dr. Francis Collins, director of the National Human Genome Research Institute, bravely tolerated each other in support of a common cause.

The occasion was the announcement of near-completion of the analysis of the entire human genetic material by the Human Genome Project (HGP), which Clinton described as "learning the language with which God created life."

Collins summed up the achievement more pragmatically as a history book with a narrative of the journey of our species through time, a shop manual with a detailed blueprint for building human beings, and "a transformative textbook of medicine."

Genetics 101

Thanks to the HGP, for the first time, nearly the whole sequence of bases that code our every characteristic and that are transmitted to our offspring was elucidated. It provided a profoundly meaningful look at that "twisted rope ladder" of the DNA molecule, whose double-helix structure was famously figured out over pints of beer in The Eagle Pub in Cambridge in 1953 by Watson and Crick.

Genes—those folded portions of the rope ladder dotted along the DNA molecule—were already known to be responsible for some diseases. But sequencing allowed much greater insight into how illnesses are caused by mutations/defects in the arrangements of those bases.

We also gained greater understanding of how a single gene defect can inevitably lead to illness, as with polycystic kidney disease, Huntington's disease, and Marfan syndrome. And we learned about how diseases so often stem from a combination of several gene defects.

Chronic and age-related conditions, like dementia and heart disease, usually involve multiple defects, for example. In type I diabetes, some thirty genes screw up many different processes, resulting in an autoimmune illness with which the immune system attacks insulin-producing islet cells in the pancreas.

These defects do not necessarily manifest immediately. Type I diabetes doesn't manifest for many years, when the pancreas finally poops out, but by then the damage is done. Also, many genetic defects don't inevitably come to pass, but increase susceptibility to illness and unhealthy environmental influences (food, pollutants, toxins, stress, etc.). Some people with defects never get sick. If you have a genetic predisposition to heart disease, for example, but eat right and keep in shape, you may never get coronary artery disease; if you spend your life on the couch chain smoking and eating bacon cheeseburgers, your predisposition may catch up with you.

A further realization, mainly attributable to the ability to sequence a genome, is that one mutation may account for more than one illness. This is often the case with cancers, as with the BRCA1 gene that predisposes to both breast and ovarian cancers. We now talk in terms of a cancer caused by a specific gene defect, rather than cancer of a specif organ.

Incidentally, mutations can be a good thing. The new DNA sequence might not make you sick, but may code for some helpful characteristic to be passed on to offspring and give them a survival advantage. This is, of course, that whole business of evolution and survival of the fittest.

The great hope of the HGP is that by knowing what's in our genetic blueprint, we'll know what to expect (predict) and how to do something about it (prevent).

Early Detection

The sooner you detect a genetic defect the better. If you can intervene in cases of juvenile diabetes before kids' pancreases give out, that's good.

Newborns are an obvious target for early detection measures. We've already been detecting genetic defects causing a variety of metabolic disorders by taking blood samples from newborns. It's a noisy business, with lab techs sticking stylettes in the heels of infants who scream bloody murder. But in this way, we detect things like phenylketonuria (PKU), thyroid disorders, and cystic fibrosis.

But even earlier is even better. Analyzing DNA before birth holds intriguing possibilities. We do some prenatal screening for things like spina bifida and Down's syndrome by taking samples of amniotic fluid or placental blood samples. But this is not without risks, including of causing a miscarriage.

Genomics can help, since sequencing requires only a minute DNA sample. It's been possible to sequence fragments of fetal DNA that leak from the fetal to the maternal circulation, which can be obtained via a regular blood sample from the mother.

This sometimes presents a tough question. If there's a problem in a developing fetus, "the couple would be faced with the dilemma of whether or not to terminate," notes the HGP website.

And now we're going even further back down the line with PGD, or pre-implantation genetic diagnosis.

This sequences cells from a newly fertilized ovum. To date, this has only been possible with in-vitro fertilization, when there's access to the fertilized ovum before implantation. But, in due course, we should be able to sequence normally fertilized ova.

This is likely to be even more fraught with ethical dilemmas and temptations to practice eugenics. Already the HGP website says, rather ominously, we can "select only mutation-free embryos."

Reservations

We may think we've learned the language with which we were created, but we're still speaking pidgin. There are plenty of questions about correct interpretation and the significance of abnormalities found during DNA analysis. And, for now at least, it's highly unlikely your doctor can tell you much about what your analysis means.

Physician and biotechnology consultant Hugh Rienhoff has a daughter with an obscure heart abnormality. Frustrated by the difficulty of getting meaningful interpretations of genome analysis related to heart problems, he set up a website, MyDaughtersDNA.org.

In a rather uncharitable mode, he offers the salutary comment that "Cardiologists don't know dog shit about genetics." This surely applies to primary care doctors as well.

As mentioned, sickness is more than just having some funky DNA. It's an interaction between your genes and the environment, and how your genes behave. Whether they are turned on or off and exactly what effects they have is controlled by epigenetics.

Epigenetics involves the portion of the DNA between the genes, unflatteringly called "junk DNA" before anyone knew its function. Now, we believe this has a lot to do with whether you succumb to your crappy diet, pollution, toxins, radiation, stress, and all the stuff that's trying to get to you.

So, you still have to listen to your doctor carping on about how you need to "eat right, exercise, don't smoke, drink in moderation," etc. Your future isn't exclusively preordained by your ancestry/genome.

And vice versa. You aren't immune to illness if your genome doesn't show any particular abnormality.

Commenting on an editorial about a recent Johns Hopkins study of the genomes of identical twins published in April 2012, the website ScitechStory notes the researchers were "outspoken about the failure of personal genomic analysis to identify a person's risk for most common diseases." People shouldn't uncritically accept negative genome findings and think they don't have to take care of themselves.

Interestingly, epigenetic influences sometimes manifest in later generations, in your children or even your grandchildren. People who smoke cigarettes in their youth affect the age of puberty of their grandchildren. The grandchildren of women malnourished during WWII in Holland were born smaller, even though their mothers were not malnourished.

Mutations also occur after genome sequencing. These can lead to problems—cancers in particular—cropping up after you've had your DNA analyzed and been cleared of certain predispositions. You can be mistaken about the hand you think you were dealt.

Do You Want To Know?

Even if you can understand what it all means, do you really want to know?

If you have something bad like the gene for incurable Huntington's Disease, which inevitably causes a very unpleasant illness with progressive neurological degeneration, writhing involuntary movements, severe emotional disturbances, and cognitive decline until you finally die over the course of a decade or two, you might not want to know.

Similarly, parents can become flipped out and overprotective if their child's genomics show some abnormality or predisposition. This is known as "vulnerable child syndrome," reports Mark Rothstein, a bioethecist at the University of Louisville.

Harvard psychologist Steven Pinker writes in *The New York Times Magazine* that "All of us already live with the knowledge that we have the fatal genetic condition called mortality, and most of us cope using some combination of denial, resignation and religion."

The idea is that getting sequenced allows you to modify your lifestyle and practice intensified surveillance (being diligent about getting your colonoscopies, mammograms, cholesterol tests, blood pressure measurements, etc). Or, you may go for more drastic preventions, as Angelina Jolie did when she got a prophylactic double mastectomy upon learning she has the BRCA1 gene (and she reportedly plans to have her ovaries removed, too).

Conversely, finding that your genome doesn't have some fatal flaw can relieve anxiety, especially if you have a specific illness that runs in your family that you've been fretting about.

Who Should Get Tested?

To offer some guidance on what—if any—testing to get done, the CDC's Office of Public Health Genomics established the Evaluation of Genomic Applications in Practice and Prevention (EGAPP, at www.egappreviews.org/default.htm). This provides advice on whether testing is valid for a variety of conditions and provides links to many other sites.

The U.S. Preventive Task Force (www.uspreventiveservices-taskforce.org) is also in on the act, releasing recommendations for "specific genetic tests used in selected clinical scenarios," like breast and colorectal cancer.

The World Health Organization and the Institute of Medicine make some testing recommendations. The advice is specific to newborns, but seems more widely applicable. It advises only getting tested "if the genetic disorder is serious and the test accurate," and only if "therapy or interventions are available."

If your racial group is vulnerable to some particular malady (like African origin predisposing to sickle cell anemia or Ashkanazi Jews being at greater risk of Tay-Sachs disease and breast cancer), that may be a reason to get tested.

If you have a family member with a genetic disease and relatives want to get tested, let the person with the illness get tested first to determine which genes are relevant. This allows for better focus during the relatives' genome examinations.

Who Else Wants To Know?

Your genomic blueprint may be of interest to others besides you. Your employer and insurance company have a keen interest in what illnesses you're likely to develop. Once the cat's out of the bag and this is in your record, it may be impossible to keep it from them.

Anticipating the potential problems, Congress, with uncommon concern for the little people, preempted any prejudice by passing the Genetic Information Nondiscrimination Act in April 2008. Ted Kennedy called it "the first major new civil rights bill of the new century." It prohibits jacking up premiums, denying coverage, or making hiring and firing decisions based on a person's genetic makeup.

TREATMENT BY GENOMICS

The obvious question is, "When we find a genetic defect, what can we do about it?" This is where the utility comes in. Can we replace the faulty gene? Can we at least do something to counteract it? Can we block the chemical path by which the faulty gene is manifesting?

We can do all of these.

Revolutions In Oncology

Cancers are often caused by defective genes, and sometimes several. If you correct or inactivate those genes, you can provide some dramatic treatments.

Traditional cancer treatment is kind of a blunderbuss therapy that kills off all rapidly dividing cells. So, not only does it kill the cancer, but it also attacks your hair, nails, and, more importantly, bone marrow. You may think of bone marrow as more of a dog food ingredient than a vital bodily organ, but it is literally your lifeblood, generating 500 billion blood cells a day and essential to many things, including oxygen transport, immunity, and blood clotting.

Finding a dose that kills the cancer but not the patient is a delicate business, so anything that enables a treatment directed at just the fault causing the cancer is an exciting idea.

As with so many cancers, multiple factors can lead to breast cancer. But one, associated with a particularly aggressive cancer, is when the cancer is HER2-positive.

A mutation of the breast cells leads to excessive production of human epidermal growth factor receptor 2 (HER2). This protein is normally present in small quantities and functions as a receptor on the cell surface. In women with HER2-positive breast cancer, this protein is present in excess, which is associated with uncontrolled reproduction of the cell. That's what cancer is: continued growth, unrestrained by those normal factors that keep cell growth in check.

Identification of this genetic fault allowed for development of a medicine called trastuzumab (marketed as Herceptin), which is a form of antibody. It seeks out and blocks the HER2 receptor. The usual analogy of an antibody attaching to a receptor is a key and lock, as an antibody is specific to a given receptor. The key fits into the lock and blocks it. The process inactivates the cancer cell and summons immune cells to take it out.

Herceptin trials showed it to be highly effective. The news got out and everyone wanted it, and there was a bit of a riot because it wasn't available outside the trial because it hadn't yet received FDA approval. This is just one of several treatment breakthroughs brought on by an understanding of genetics and made possible by the genome project and related research.

Of interest is that the same genetic abnormality can affect different tissues. Like breast cancer, stomach cancer can also be associated with elevated HER2. This realization changes the perspective away from an organ-specific disease to a gene-specific disease.

This has implications for the drug approval process. If a drug has been approved to treat HER2 disease of the breast, it's questionable whether new clinical trials should be mandated for the same medicine to treat HER2 stomach cancer.

In the case of colon cancer, the FDA redeemed themselves some. The story, which is much like the HER2 story, illustrates another benefit of genetics in cancer care.

Colon cancer is another serious player in the cancer field. Colorectal cancer is the third most common, with about 140,000 new cases annually, according to the American Cancer Society. Just how mean and nasty is it? At least 50,000 of those patients die.

Colon cancer cells have receptors called epidermal growth factor receptors (EGFR), instead of HER2. I know it's confusing, with all the receptors sounding so similar, and don't ask me why there are epidermal growth factor receptors on breast and colon cells when the epidermis is part of the skin. But there's this whole family of human epidermal growth factor receptors involved in a lot of cancers.

With colon cancer, there's also a KRAS gene involved in activating the EGFRs. Sometimes, the cancer presents with a normal KRAS gene (despite the cell being cancerous), sometimes an abnormal one.

Like trastuzumab blocks the receptors in breast cancer, a drug called cetuximab (brand name Erbitux) blocks the EGFRs in colon cancer.

The catch is cetuximab doesn't work if there's a mutation in the KRAS gene. This mutation is present in 30 to 50 percent of colon cancer cases, making cetuximab/Erbitux useless for about one-third to one-half of patients.

Interestingly, doctors currently prescribe Erbitux indiscriminately in all colon cancer cases. Basically, they don't know any better, complains Paul Howard, Ph.D., director of the Manhattan Institute's Center for Medical Progress, writing on the MedicalProgressToday blog he edits.

"If it were given only to those in whom it works, the healthcare system could save up to $600 million a year," he claims.

It's now possible to use genomics to identify cancers with the KRAS mutation. In July 2009, the FDA earned a few points by updating the label of cetuximab/Erbitux (and the similar panitumumab/Vectibix) to inform doctors of the difference in efficacy based on the presence of the mutation.

GENE CORRECTION TREATMENT

The ultimate treatment, and the "most exciting application of DNA sequencing," as the HGP website puts it, is to correct a gene defect itself.

This came too late for David Vetter, the "Bubble Boy" for whom "Bubble Boy disease" is named. He had severe combined immunodeficiency disease (SCID, with which a faulty gene causes deficiency of the adenosine deaminase enzyme. This leads to immune system failure and repeated infections. Untreated, affected kids almost always die between 2 and 5 years old.

Vetter, born in 1971, became the famous exception. He was kept alive by living in a giant sterile "bubble," a sealed chamber that protected him from germs. This measure kept him going till age 12.

Traditionally, SCID is treated with donated stem cells from a bone marrow transplant which restore the body's immuno-competence. But there are lots of obstacles and complications, foremost among them finding a good donor-recipient match.

In David's case, his sister was a fairly good match, and she donated. Unfortunately, she had mononucleosis in the past and the Epstein-Barr virus was still holed up in her body. It contaminated the bone marrow transplant and the virus got the upper hand; tragically, David died fifteen days later.

A new treatment, pioneered by H. Bobby Gaspar, M.D., Ph.D., of UCL Institute of Child Health in London, uses the patient's own harvested stem cells, making them a perfect match, of course. The defective gene is replaced, ironically enough, with the help of another virus, a retrovirus. When these modified stem cells are reintroduced, they grow back and replace the faulty bone marrow, restoring the immune system.

A recent report on WebMD notes that fourteen of sixteen patients who underwent this gene replacement treatment are alive and well. "These children, who would have died," notes Dr. Gaspar, "are going to school, playing ball, and going to parties."

SCID is just one of a slew of illnesses caused by defective genes. Fixing broken genes comes with plenty of practical problems, but other diseases, like sickle cell anemia, hemophilia, thalassemia, muscular dystrophy, and cystic fibrosis, are caused by single genetic mutations and are potential candidates for this kind of treatment.

Pharmacogenomics

Genomics analysis has also affected treatment through pharmacogenomics, the branch of pharmacology that deals with the influence of genetic variation on drug response in patients.

As noted, your genes play a role in how your body responds to toxins. This includes reactions to those "toxins" we take intentionally, the ones we call medicines.

Pharmacogenomics can help to refine individualized medicine dosing; to know which medicines will work on which people, because, as with the KRAS gene story, not everyone responds to every drug; and to know who will suffer which adverse effects (a good thing to know, given that 100,000 people die every year from adverse drug reactions and many more are made ill).

Some go so far as to claim giving medicines without knowledge of the genome is like giving a blood transfusion without typing the blood first.

The story of platelet adhesion inhibitor clopidogrel is a good illustration of the benefit of knowing whom a medicine will work on.

A blood clot begins when platelets stick together. This is desirable if you cut yourself or are bleeding somewhere, but when it happens spontaneously inside a blood vessels, it can lead to a blockage and a stroke or heart attack. Aspirin helps make plate-lets less sticky, and a lot of people take a daily baby aspirin to reduce their risk (although there has been a lot of recent debate about the validity).

Clopidogrel was developed and marketed by Bristol-Myers Squibb and Sanofi Pharmaceuticals as Plavix and announced with much fanfare in August 1995, claiming it showed significant superiority to aspirin.

Eric Topol, M.D., attended the announcement and writes about the reception at the fabulously opulent Hotel de Crillon in Paris. He was distinctly unimpressed by the clinical findings, noting Plavix showed only an 8.7 percent improvement over aspirin, with only two patients per 100 benefiting.

Still, Plavix was granted "priority regulatory review," a process normally reserved for important new medicines for life-threatening conditions, and it became the second-biggest selling drug worldwide.

One way it was used was in patients with a stent (a tube placed in a diseased artery to hold it open). But stents tend to be perceived by the body as foreign objects and trigger clots, as does any foreign object in the vascular system. People were put on Plavix to reduce the risk of this happening. With time, it became apparent that it didn't work in 30 percent of patients, and they had a disastrous 300 percent increase in the risk of the stent clotting off. Unfortunately, there was no way to know who those patients would be. Until genome analysis came along.

Then it was discovered that these non-responders have an abnormality in the gene that codes for the cytochrome CYP2C19 enzyme, responsible for converting clopidogrel to a slightly different active compound in the body, which if absent meant there was no platelet inhibition.

When it became possible to identify these "non-converters," the FDA came up with a new type of black box warning, telling prescribers it won't work on some patients, who can be identified with genome analysis.

Similarly, pharmacogenomics has potential to make a huge difference in diabetes management. There are eleven different drug classes for treating diabetes, and we spend about $29 billion per year on them, relates Topol. But "We know the most commonly used drug doesn't even work in about 25 percent of patients."

Detecting Side Effects

Statin medicines, like Lipitor, Zocor, and Crestor, are taken by many people to lower cholesterol. The CDC reports that from 1999 to 2009, our overfed society saw a tenfold increase in the use of statins in some age groups.

Some people can't take them due to a genetic abnormality that causes muscle inflammation and pain with statin use. This is slightly less drastic than the story of Plavix, but a significant problem simply because of the number of people taking these drugs—including half of all American men ages 65 to 74.

Similarly, codeine (and derivatives) are in a lot of pain medicines. To work, it's converted to morphine in the body. But there's great variability in how effectively different people's metabolism make this conversion, and if you happen to be a rapid converter, it's not too hard to overdose on what would be a therapeutic dose for someone else.

Or, the severe skin reaction to the anti-seizure medicine carbamazapine (Tegretol) or the possible allergic reaction to anti-HIV medicine abacavir (Ziagen) are examples of more serious adverse effects that occur unpredictably in some people.

I once wrote about this in my monthly column for my local newspaper. I predicted the ability to do genomic testing to identify the people who can't take statins would eventually be a reality.

Just a few months later, I got a demonstration of how rapidly the field of pharmacogenomics is advancing. I was brought up short, bumbling about in our bathroom one morning listening to NPR as usual. A commercial played from Vanderbilt University Medical Center touting their available PREDICT program that allows a "doctor to use the results from the test to make better decisions about the drugs that are right for you." They were already selling this test to the public.

The field is taking off and more companies are getting in on the act. My nephew recently asked me to write an order for YouScript (www.YouScript.com) to ascertain his reaction to a bunch of medicines he takes for a weird autoimmune disease he has.

YouScript notes, "Approximately 75 percent of patients have detectable variations in their DNA which may increase their risk of an adverse drug event" and advises you get tested if you take multiple medicines, if you've had problems getting the dosage right in the past, or if you think the medicines you take aren't working.

Dosing Insights

And now, on to warfarin, aka Coumadin. It's a good example of how pharmacogenomics can help with the ticklish business of figuring out correct dosages.

You may know warfarin as a rat poison, but it's popular among people as well. The same anticoagulant properties that cause fatal hemorrhages in rodents can effectively treat and prevent blood clots in humans. However, getting the degree of anticoagulation just right requires frequent blood tests to check the "pro time" to prevent patients from going out like rats with catastrophic bleeds or developing blood clots in spite of treatment.

The risk is not insubstantial. Currently, 2 to 10 percent of patients have bleeds in the first year of treatment and 1 percent of them die, usually from strokes. It's often necessary to go to the trouble and expense of having special Coumadin clinics to monitor patients on anticoagulants.

Couple the inherent risks and the need for diligent monitoring with the fact that many patients on warfarin are old, confused, or unreliable. Thankfully, genome sequencing has revealed several genetic variations and made warfarin dosing a lot more precise and safer. Granted, there's a rather complicated dosing chart depending on whether you have one or more of the genetic variations affecting metabolism of warfarin, but it's progress. Progress that saves lives.

CHANGES TO CLINICAL TRIALS

The evolution of genomics and pharmacogenomics will undoubtedly force changes to the FDA's rules for getting drugs to market.

The present clinical trial system is very much a one-size-fits-all endeavor. The same dose of the trial medicine is given to thousands or hundreds of thousands of subjects for years. The researchers wait and see what happens.

But, as mentioned above with the HER2-positive cancers, in the future, studies will increasingly deal with treatments that help a particular genetic defect. Things are going to be "overtaken rapidly by patients who know their own genomes," predicts Topol. They and the pharmaceutical companies won't be content to go through laborious decade-long clinical trials that cost billions of dollars.

Barbara Bradfield, a 48-year-old from Burbank, California, had HER2 breast cancer. Oncologist, researcher, and writer Siddhartha Mukherjee described her case in his book *The Emperor of All Maladies*. It's a good illustration of the conflicts developing.

Bradfield was treated with bilateral mastectomy and seven months of chemo, but the cancer relapsed. She said she was "at the end of my road" and had "accepted what seemed inevitable."

Meanwhile, while working for bioengineering company Gentech, oncologist and researcher Dennis Slamon had developed an antibody to the HER2 gene. It had only been tried *in vitro* and in mice, but he was starting a clinical trial.

Slamon reviewed Bradfield's slides and called her unexpectedly. He told her she had one of the highest levels of HER2 he'd ever seen and that she'd be an ideal candidate for the trial. At first she refused, but Slamon persisted and talked her into it.

In the four months between his asking and the start of the trial, Bradfield developed a lump in her neck and sixteen new masses in her lungs. Mukherjee describes how the women in the trial had become a close-knit group and carefully followed each other's progress. They all palpated the lumps in Bradfield's neck every time they got together for the next round of treatment.

A few months into the trial, all the women agreed the lump in her neck were much smaller, as were her lung metastases. Bradfield completed a total of eighteen months of therapy. After resigning herself to the inevitability of an early death from cancer, Bradfield is still alive today.

News of the seemingly miraculous success spread. Breast cancer activists "pounded on Gentech's door," notes Mukherjee, urging the release of the drug to women with HER2-positive cancers in whom other treatments failed. Many, in desperation, were willing to risk "compassionate use" of a relatively untried medicine. The activists argued the women "could not wait for the drug to undergo interminable testing."

But "Gentech wanted carefully executed, early phase trials." The company would not provide the drug even for compassionate use to patients who would otherwise inevitably die.

This is a tricky issue that's arisen before. When someone comes up with a particularly successful treatment, everyone understandably wants it right away, but that screws up the statistical proof of its efficacy.

Consider the rest of the trastuzumab/Herceptin story. It took a decade of testing for it to be approved by the FDA in 2010 for use in patients with HER2 stomach cancer.

Commenting on this difficult issue, Topol says, "We have this big thing about evidence-based medicine and, of course, the sanctimonious, randomized, placebo-controlled clinical trial." But when a product has been developed to fix a targeted defect—and especially when there is no alternative available—the FDA protocol of a years-long placebo-controlled trial with half the patients taking a sugar pill is a hard sell, Topol elaborates. "We need a different position at the FDA."

There are also non-genomic "future" factors likely to affect clinical trials. In particular, improved post-marketing surveillance via computerized medical records and health information systems makes for much more efficient identification of adverse drug reactions. We saw it with Kaiser's computerized medical records catching on to heart attacks in patients taking Vioxx (as mentioned in *Getting the Right Treatment*).

Things may be improving for people hoping to get their hands on new, potentially life-saving medicines. In the summer of 2012, with large bipartisan support, Congress passed the FDA Safety and Innovation Act. Part of this act helps speed up the approval process of new medicines, especially ones for "serious or life-threatening conditions," notes an October 2012 Perspective on the *New England Journal of Medicine* website.

Ten Years After The HGP

Extravagant claims have been made for the benefit of genomics in medicine. "Doctors will be able to diagnose many illnesses instantly and target them with designer drugs" and "Eventually scientists will be able to model and mold the incredibly complex interaction between genes and the environment that determines physical and mental health, or disease over the life span," predicts psychologist and author Robert E. Adler.

But this smacks of the hubris the medical profession is so good at and reminiscent of past claims of imminent extinction of disease that tend to accompany groundbreaking advances like antibiotics, vaccinations, and anesthetics. In fact, ten years after the fanfare upon completion of the Human Genome Project, it seems the excitement, novelty, and hopes have faded a bit.

What if a patient doesn't have a specific genetic defect that can be identified or corrected? What if a patient doesn't have some issue pharmacogenomics can tailor a medicine to? It all still comes down to old-fashioned lifestyle modifications and conventional surveillance, getting your mammogram or colonoscopy, getting off the couch, getting off the *Super Size Me* diet and cigarettes... the usual stuff you've heard over and over.

But perhaps these measures can be tweaked and focused in light of what a person's genome indicates susceptibility to. At high risk for Alzheimers? Take up Sudoku and maintain an active social life. Prone to colon cancer? Early detection makes a big difference in the prognosis, so get frequent fecal occult blood tests and colonoscopies.

The problem with this approach is invariably human foibles—the limited ability or willingness of people to be diligent. A review ten years after completion of the HGP was a bit disappointing, in large part because most people don't have some correctable defect. They are left trying to stave off any illnesses they've been found susceptible to with good behavior.

The Scripps Health Initiative performed a study of 3,600 individuals sequenced with a Navigenics scan. Findings indicate increased risk of various illnesses, especially different kinds of cancers. "No clear evidence of lifestyle improvement" or of people taking heed of their increased risks by undergoing appropriate screenings was found, laments Topol.

DNA FINGERPRINTING

Individual "spelling mistakes" (more properly called single nucleotide polymorphisms, or SNPs) in an organism's genome sequence, which are passed on to offspring, provide a way of establishing a unique identity.

This is used already in DNA "fingerprinting" and in tracing ancestry/evolution. The company 23andMe, probably the best known of the many companies offering this service, offers a limited analysis for a modest $299. They will trace your lineage back "10,000 years and beyond," they say, and tell you how Neanderthal you are.

The sample used for sequencing is usually a buccal smear, taken from the inside of your cheek with a cotton swab. You only need a tiny fragment of tissue containing DNA to analyze. It even allows for identification of old or badly decomposed bodies, as with the body dug up in a parking lot in Leicester, England being identified as the long-lost Richard III via a fragment of DNA from a tooth.

Medically, this is a method for better compatibility testing between transplant donors and recipients and for tracing the source of nasty infections.

Recently, a team in Cambridge, England was investigating a recurrent outbreak of the dreaded "superbug" methicillin-resistant *Staphylococcus aureus* (MRSA) in the local hospital's Special Care Baby Unit that had struck twelve infants in six months. It hadn't proven possible to trace the source with traditional antibiotic susceptibility profiles. But with whole genome sequencing of the bacterial DNA, the researchers were able to show that the infections were linked and being passed back and forth between mothers in the SCBU, the maternity ward, and the community.

It's reminiscent of Semmelweis proving "childbed fever" (peurpural sepsis) was caused by microbes transmitted from infected patients to new ones by doctors not washing their hands between the mortuary and the delivery ward.

Identifying uniquely patterned SNPs is also used to establish parenthood in paternity suits and the like. Now there are even DIY kits.

COMMERCIALIZATION AND REGULATION

The possibility that genomics can reveal your or your child's sporting, artistic, or intellectual capabilities; who you're likely to get along with romantically; what diet suits you; your ancestry; and what medical issues may overtake you in the future makes genome sequencing an intriguing business and an appealing commodity with great sales potential.

The entrepreneurs have dived right in, and hundreds of companies offer sequencing services. It's already gotten to the point where regulators are taking interest.

In 2008, *TIME* deemed retail genomics the top invention of the year. But some complain that the FDA is being a bit of a spoilsport. In 2010, it nixed Walgreens' plans to market a Pathway Genomics testing kit, on the grounds it was considered a medical device and as such had to be approved by the agency first. In November 2013, it told 23andMe they had to stop telling people about their predispositions to ninety medical conditions "from baldness to blindness," as this qualified as a medical device (the company still analyzes ancestry and provides raw data on genomic make up, but doesn't interpret potentially medically significant findings).

The technology is predictably advancing and dropping in price. In an interview in *AARP Bulletin* in March 2014, Francis Collins notes you can now get sequenced "for around $1,000, which is amazing given that it cost $400 million 10 years ago."

It's also getting faster. Pacific Bioscience predicts their second-generation machine, due for release in 2015, will do a full sequence in fifteen minutes for $100. Genomics for the masses.

Last Word

Genome sequencing is still an imperfect science. What regulations the FDA will impose is still a moot issue. The technology still isn't fully refined. Interpretation is still iffy even in the best hands, and I doubt most people's primary care doctor will be much help when they bring their gene maps.

But in true medically emancipated style, you can order and interpret for yourself. Many companies offer sequencing (23andMe, FamilyTreeDNA, Ancestry.com, Complete Genomics, etc.). Some have sections to help you interpret results, and separate sites exist specifically for interpretation (like diygenomics. pbworks.com). But it's all pretty technical stuff, and as Topol reports, "The American Medical Association has lobbied the government hard for consumers not to have direct access to their genomic data."

Writing online in *Upstart Business Journal* about getting genome sequencing done by several different companies, journalist David Ewing Duncan notes one company told him he needed statins immediately to stave off heart disease while another said he was at decreased risk of heart disease.

I discussed recommended criteria to help decide whether you should get sequenced, but I like the quote from *Jurassic Park* about how "Our scientists were so preoccupied with whether they could, they didn't stop to think if they should."

Undoubtedly, many claims from the sequencing companies are a bit hyped. But it's a highly technical, rapidly evolving field, which gives me reservations about being competent to tell you all about it and it not being outdated by the time you read it. There's no question, though, that genomics can tell you fascinating stuff about your personal proclivities, ancestry, and health expectations.

CREATURES OF THE MICROBIOME

Even after sequencing the entire human genome, the NIH wasn't ready to call it quits. After HGP, they launched the Human Microbiome Project (HMP) to explore a hot new area of interest in medicine. The "microbiome" refers to the whole mess of microorganisms living in and on our body. It includes some 10,000 species of cooties.

You may have an "eeewwww" moment at the thought of all these critters (bacteria, viruses, yeasts, and obscure microorganisms like helminths, eukarytes, and archaea) living in your nose, sinuses, skin, belly button, vagina, intestines, and other nooks and crannies.

But these organisms do a lot of good by breaking down food to molecules small enough to metabolize, manufacturing products like vitamin K that we can't produce for ourselves, detoxifying poisons, shielding our skin and intestines against competing pathogenic organisms that try to establish there, and helping our immune system. The latter function is likely significant in immune-mediated/inflammatory GI diseases, like Crohn's and ulcerative colitis, and possibly even beyond (there's speculation the breakdown of insulating myelin in nerves in multiple sclerosis may be due to an immune response related to the microbiome of the gut).

Our microbiome possesses hundreds of times as much genetic materials as our bodies do, and these genes seem to interact with and regulate our own genes. In terms of comparative cell count, there are nine "cootie" cells to every one of ours. So, you could argue we are more microbiome than human, and some use the term "holobionts" for this mutually beneficial genetic interaction.

Barnett Kramer, M.D., M.P.H., director of the division of cancer prevention at the National Cancer Institute, thinks the principal gains go to the microorganisms, though. We benefit from having them on board, he says, but "we may just serve as packaging."

The HMP was headed up by Dr. Francis Collins, who described this new project as "like 15th century explorers describing the outline of a new continent."

Previous attempts to analyze the microbiome were foiled because many of the organisms are too fastidious to grow in conventional culture. But new genome sequencing allowed exact identification of the different critters by taking samples from the noses, mouths, skin, stool, and vaginas of 242 healthy adults and painstakingly analyzing the DNA over five years, at a cost of $153 million. It was a field day for geneticists, as there are some 360 times more genes as in the human genome.

We've developed this relationship with microorganisms throughout our evolution. Even creatures as primitive as jellyfish have microbiomes. But every newborn is pristine in the mother's sterile womb, until the puling infant starts that traumatic journey through the profuse microflora of the vagina. But this isn't as awful as it sounds. Researchers from Baylor College of Medicine in Houston found that the microbiome of a woman's vagina alters radically just before birth, reducing the number of species present. After birth, the infant "is a bacterial sponge, as it populates its own microbiome," notes the NIH News website.

The significance of the microbiome is indicated by some findings of babies born by C-section. Obviously, they aren't exposed to the vaginal flora, and often suffer the further "benefit" of the mother's prophylactic antibiotic shot. Plus, C-section mothers often can't or are discouraged from breastfeeding, which also seems to be significant in the formation of a newborn's microbiome.

As reported in the *Canadian Medical Association Journal*, these babies seem to have a different microbiome and an increased risk for allergies, asthma, diabetes, and other chronic conditions.

We are "working on better understanding the effects that these changes on the gut bacteria have on long-term health," says Meghan Azad, Ph.D., assistant professor of pediatrics and child health at the University of Manitoba.

Research is focusing on whether we need to reverse our "clean-freak" mentality and whether we're being overzealous with our hygiene and avoiding microorganisms. It's also looking at whether manipulation of the microbiome by deliberately introducing normal miroorganisms (bacteria, mostly) helps prevent some problems like allergies, a host of autoimmune illness like lupus and type 1 diabetes, mental disorders like autism and schizophrenia, and even obesity and dandruff.

It also seems in our naivety we tend to disregard the importance of our microbiome with our profligate use of antibiotics, which wipe out the good microorganisms along with the pathogens.

Consider overgrowth of resistant *Clostridium difficile* bacteria, which results from screwing with the normal intestinal flora with administration of antibiotics. It causes life-threatening diarrhea and damage from pseudomembranous colitis that affects 3 million people per year in the U.S. and kills 14,000.

Cutting-edge research is focusing on ways to correct these transgressions. Medically emancipated patient Catherine Duff is a trailblazer on this front.

She was literally dying of *C. difficile* colitis, caused by antibiotics from her dentist, despite multiple treatment attempts. She was at the point where her surgeon told her "the easiest thing to do" was remove her colon and get a colostomy bag attached to her abdominal wall to collect stool.

With the help of her daughter, she found out about Dr. Thomas Brody in Australia who'd been doing fecal microbiota transplantation (FMT) for some twenty years. It involves introducing a slurry of healthy stool into the intestine to restore a healthy microbiome.

The procedure was referred to less properly on *Grey's Anatomy* as a "poop transplant." But Duff couldn't get any of her U.S. doctors to do it. "These physicians ... were denied permission to perform FMT by their practice partners or affiliated hospitals ... citing liability concerns," she said in an interview.

With the help of her husband, she infused herself by enema with a sample of healthy donor stool. Within a mere six hours, she felt a whole lot better and proceeded to recover from there.

A Dutch study of the procedure (which did not give control subjects Nutella as a placebo, as one comedian suggested on Twitter) was so successful, with over 80 percent cured with a single infusion, it was stopped early.

Since then, this has become a recognized method of treatment for severe and stubborn cases of *C. diff* colitis and is being tried for constipation, general colitis, irritable bowel syndrome, and even multiple sclerosis.

Probiotics is another relatively new way of keeping your microbiome healthy. These are doses of beneficial bacteria. They're naturally occurring in some foods, like yogurt, sauerkraut, and kimchi, and available in fortified foods and supplements. Their action can be enhanced with prebiotics (nondigestible carbohydrates that stimulate growth and/or activity of bacteria in the GI tract). Prebiotics and probiotics can be taken together to potentate each other; yogurt conveniently supplies both.

Probiotics have been enthusiastically embraced by people into natural remedies, which of course they are. It would appear they can do more than fix GI problems, reducing colds, helping allergies, lowering LDL (bad) cholesterol, and reducing dental decay. Undoubtedly we'll discover additional benefits as we learn more about the microbiome.

We now "understand what the normal human microbiome looks like," says Barbara Methé, Ph.D., of the J. Craig Venter Institute in Rockville, Maryland. We "should be able to understand how changes in the microbiome are associated with, or even cause, illnesses," too.

There's still much to learn about this rose garden within us, with its own massive composite genome.

REGENERATIVE MEDICINE

Regenerative medicine, or the artificial growth of new tissues and organs to replace and repair damaged or diseased ones, is another futuristic business greatly helped along by genomics and the ability to analyze and tinker with DNA.

Normally, cells are programmed to develop into a particular tissue or organ. Heart muscle cells make more heart tissue, nerve cells make nerves, and liver cells make liver, explains Anthony Atala, M.D., director of the Wake Forest Institute for Regenerative Medicine.

But now, with the right culture conditions or by manipulating genetic material, we can transform any kind of cells into any other, "if only researchers can prod them into action," says Atala.

Conveniently, this sidesteps the need for unused fertilized cells from in vitro fertilization, which have the capability of growing into human beings. Their use is controversial, with concerns about "personhood" and sentimentality about human life.

So far, it's been possible to grow bone, cartilage, corneas, tracheas, arteries, urethras, and more. Cultured heart muscle has been injected into mice with heart failure and improved cardiac function. Recently, researcher Douglas Melton (who has two children with diabetes) and a team from Harvard University announced they had used stem cell technology to grow billions of insulin-secreting cells, pointing to the exciting possibility of curing type I diabetes. And Japanese scientists have gone so far as to produce ova that have been fertilized and created apparently normal offspring.

The possibility of growing nerve cells holds particular promise. Nerves typically don't repair themselves, or do so incredibly slowly, so this could be a game-changer for people with degenerative neurological conditions like Parkinson's, ALS, or crippling spinal cord injuries.

There's also the potential to grow whole limbs, which has caught the attention of the military. It's invested $85 million, creating the Armed Forces Institute for Regenerative Medicine in partnership with Wake Forest University, inspired in part by the story of Lee Spievack.

As reported by various sources, Spievack cut off the tip of his finger with the propeller of a model airplane. His brother, conveniently enough working in the field of tissue regeneration, sent him some "pixie dust" of protein and connective tissue derived from pig bladders, similar to that used to help tendons mend.

Within four weeks, Spievack's finger had regenerated all components and completely grown back, though skeptics claim it wasn't such a significant injury and would have done fine with conventional therapy. Still, the story generated interest and intrigue, and the military hopes to eventually pull the same trick for entire limbs of injured/amputee soldiers.

GROWING ORGANS

Organs are either a solid mass of tissue cells or they grow over some kind of "scaffold." There's currently much research being done on manufacturing whole organs.

The Karolinska Institute in Sweden is pioneering the field, though with a lot of international cooperation. One of the first subjects was a 36 year old needing a new trachea. Earlier attempts at tracheal transplant used donated cadaver tracheas with all cellular material removed and then recolonized with cultured cells. But a recent advance has been to form the scaffold out of biodegradable material like polymers or collagen.

This was done at Karolinska in June 2011, with a scaffold made of a nano-composite supplied by University College, London, and colonized with the patient's own stem cells, grown for two days prior to implantation in a bioreactor from Harvard Bioscience. The process was a great success.

Innovations in 3D printing are facilitating organ manufacturing. It's a source of serious excitement in many fields, despite concerns among non-NRA members about hoodlums printing off the lower receivers of guns.

Using an MRI or CT to provide an image to copy, 3D printing can lay down layers of polymer or collagen to make an organ's scaffold. Or, as done by San Diego-based company Organovo, the cultured cells themselves can be used as "ink" to build whole organs layer by layer.

Atala has built miniature kidneys this way that function and produce urine. He's also pioneered growing new bladders, as he did for Luke Masella, a child with spina bifida whose kidneys were being destroyed because of his malfunctioning bladder.

At 10, Masella received a new bladder grown by Atala. He joined Atala on stage at a recent conference as a showpiece of success, a healthy, active sophomore at the University of Connecticut.

Perhaps soon you'll be able to walk into Kinkos for copies of your holiday card photos and a replacement of whatever organ you're not entirely happy with.

The ability to manufacture tissues and organs may be a huge boon to the many desperate people on transplant waiting lists. And the ability to turn any individual adult cells into effective stem cells is likely to eliminate the other primary pitfall, finding a donor who is immunologically a good match.

Grown tissues cultures also allows for testing drugs at a cellular level.

Hopefully, this will replace a lot of pharmaceutical animal testing during early stages of development. It's less likely to call down the condemnation of animal rights activists if a drug company poisons a few cells rather than a bunch of bunny rabbits or puppies.

Winnowing down viable pharmaceuticals is an inefficient business; in 2011, nearly 900 anti-cancer medicines and vaccines were in clinical trials, yet only 12 oncology drugs were approved by the FDA that year. But "Cancer treatments are being increasingly tailored to target particular genetic variants," notes an article in *Nature*. Cell cultures allow multiple samples of the same genetic makeup, which can be used in the screening process.

Also, growing cells into types of tissues we can't take samples of without doing harm (like arteries or nerve cells) allows testing at a cellular level that previously wasn't possible. At the Salk Institute, for example, researchers have been using cell cultures to see what effects different drugs have on the defective nerve cells of schizophrenics.

IMAGING

Until we evolve enough to master predict-and-prevent health-care, imaging is an essential tool. It's currently undergoing rapid change, making us more and more like that bizarre plastic toy, the "Visible Man," whom you can see right through.

X-Ray

In 1895, German physicist Conrad Rontgen discovered penetrating rays with which he could image his wife's hand. It wasn't until X-rays were used with abandon, even in shoe shops, that the toxicity of this ionizing radiation became apparent, perhaps vindicating Frau Roentgen's comment on seeing the image of her bones: "I have seen my death."

Digital radiology, which captures images electronically instead of on large, cumbersome, celluloid photographic film, is a useful advance. It's been widely adopted for mammography, reducing radiation exposure and allowing for image manipulation on a computer to view it from all angles. Plus, the computer sifts through the zillions of images created and highlights the suspect ones.

These images can be viewed wherever you have a computer (my medical group was recently negotiating with a group of radiologists in Australia to read our films). So, radiologists no longer have to drag their sorry asses out of bed in the middle of the night to go into the hospital for some train wreck in the ER; they only need to open up their laptops.

CT Scanners

With EMI's massive earnings from the Beatles, the company invented the CT scanner. This allowed for revealing images comprised of tomographic "slices" piled into 3D pictures. Resolution has improved from the original sixteen-slice images to 256-slice pictures with which we can detect atheroma on the inside of coronary arteries or developing cancers inside the colon with virtual colonoscopy.

CT scanners have also become fast enough to image whole bodies to detect injuries when people are sufficiently beaten up that they can't indicate where they hurt. The technology has also made it feasible for the military to scan every conscript to provide a baseline image on their futuristic thumb drive dog tags (mentioned in *Getting the Right Information*).

They've been used for autopsies, too. The British Museum used CT imaging to determine a several thousand-year-old mummy likely died of stab wounds.

Further detail can be obtained with injected or imbibed substances that create a contrast in radiographic density between different tissues, but still there's the drawback of using ionizing radiation.

MRI Scanners

When mathematician and physician Raymond V. Damadian figured out how to make a very nice image from the radiation emitted by the nuclei of cells exposed to a strong magnetic field, the MRI scanner got us away from those toxic rays.

This provided better resolution than CTs, but still only showed structure.

The buzz these days is imaging techniques that also indicate function. With a little tinkering, it's been possible to modify MRI images according to the amount of oxygen in the blood. This can show metabolic activity of the tissue, and the functional MRI, or fMRI, was born.

Brain imaging with fMRI can indicate abnormal function in various pathologies and offers hope in helping with Alzheimer's, Parkinson's, autism, schizophrenia, ADD, and other conditions. It can even tell if someone's lying or whether an advertisement effectively lights up the pleasure centers.

A further development was spectroscopy, which detects different chemical constituents in tissues, providing various diagnostic benefits. For example, it shows the metabolites of inflammation in many diseases, including atheroma (providing another means of detecting crud buildup in blood vessels), and it detects choline, a nutrient found in elevated levels in breast and prostate cancer.

One particular hope of MRI spectroscopy is that it will help with the tricky problem of young women who have small, dense breasts. They might look great to fashion designers, but they're notoriously difficult to image with standard mammography.

PET Scanners

In 1953, the seven-year-old daughter of a Rhode Island farmer developed a mystery neurological illness that stopped her from being able to read and left her staring vacantly. Conventional diagnostic and imaging methods drew a blank.

She was referred to Massachusetts General Hospital, where Dr. Gordon L. Brownell and others were using imaging with positron-emitting radioactive glucose tracers. Positron emission tomography, or PET scans, which show variations in the metabolic rate of rapidly reproducing cancer cells, revealed that the girl had a brain tumor with sufficient accuracy (within one-third of an inch) to allow successful removal.

PET scanners are particularly good at detecting cancers. They're used to find the primary cancer source of peripheral metastases, for staging by determining where the cancer has spread, and to assess the efficacy of treatment.

Scans can be improved with radionuclides, showing promise for detecting Alzheimer's, neurological foci of seizures, psychiatric diseases, and possibly even substance abuse. They can also detect "hibernating" myocardium, an area of heart muscle much less metabolically active because of deficient blood supply, indicating blocked coronary arteries.

Psychiatrist Gary Small, M.D., director of UCLA's Longevity Center at the Semel Institute for Neuroscience & Human Behavior, has used markers attached to tau proteins (which appear to be indicative of concussion) to document the damage Neanderthals do to each other playing football.

PET scans may also help pharmaceutical development with their ability to measure distribution and elimination of drugs.

ULTRASOUND

This technology, stolen from bats and dolphins, was used to locate the Titanic and later enemy submarines. It uses high-frequency sounds to create an image, and it's popular because it's cheap, safe (actually therapeutic in some instances), and mobile.

Fetal "sonograms" are probably the most familiar application, with the ability to make "truly beautiful images of the unborn baby," says Stephen C. Schimpff, M.D.

It's spawned a whole industry around letting you "Watch in amazement and gleam with happiness as your blessed miracle begins to suck on their fingers and toes, yawn, twist and turn," as the gushing advertisement for InfantSee4D puts it. This is one of many companies that, for a fee of around $300, allows you and up to ten family members to spend up to thirty minutes watching your unborn baby thrash around. Some—including these companies, to be sure—claim this enhances bonding and encourages mothers to forgo any unhealthy habits during pregnancy.

But it's not just for fun and voyeurism. Fetal sonograms are invaluable to doctors, as is the ability to image most body parts or places a creative doctor can think to stick an ultrasound probe. For example, transesophageal ultrasounds get close to the heart, rectal ultrasounds look at structures of the bowel or prostate, and transvaginal ultrasounds explore the pelvis and uterine contents (including the controversial mandate in some states that this be used on women seeking an abortion).

Imaging the heart (echocardiogram) has been done for a long time, showing the structure of valves and other parts and assessing the efficiency of the heart's contractions. The quality and resolution of ultrasound machines is rapidly increasing, while size and price are decreasing, so instead of "a $300,000 machine the size of a refrigerator" used at a cost of $1,500, notes cardiologist Topol, we have machines like the Vscan. They're small enough to fit in a white coat pocket and are replacing stethoscopes, often obviating the need to send the patient for a formal echocardiogram.

Ultrasound can also be enhanced. One technique uses microbubble contrast, with a bunch of tiny bubbles better reflecting the ultrasound waves. This can show detail like the microcirculation of tumors and other pathologies like cirrhosis in the liver. It can even be further refined for some organ imaging by attaching chemical "hooks" to the bubbles.

The technology shows promise for one particularly troublesome issue: differentiating sinister from benign moles (or "nevi," to be more clinically correct). Trying to figure this out has probably been the most fly-by-the-seat-of-your-pants aspect of modern medicine. The ability of high frequency ultrasound to differentiate could save doctors a lot of sleepless nights. And a lot of lives.

And while on the subject of dermatological imaging and the war against the worrisome rise in melanoma, there's also a doodad that emits rays in the terahertz range (between microwave and infrared) that can be read with a smartphone camera. It sees beneath superficial layers and can "more accurately and almost instantaneously diagnose melanoma," reports PCMag.com.

OPTICAL IMAGING AND MORE

One particular technique—optical imaging—may bring some color and joy back into the life of my interventional radiologist friend John, who spends a lot of time sitting in his dark, dreary, monochrome world in the gloomy hospital basement reading X-rays (it's a good thing he gets paid so much).

This technology uses diffusion and absorption of near-infrared light from a laser probe, creating an image that provides information about molecular structure, metabolic activity, and blood flow. It can be improved with the addition of fluorescent dyes, producing spectacular psychedelic images.

Optical imaging is already used in pulse oximeters, those things with the red light they clamp onto your finger in the doctor's office, OR, and ER to measure oxygenation. It also shows promise for deciding whether a breast lump is cancerous without biopsy; for making sure the wound margins are clear when resecting a cancer; for identifying plaque in the arteries—especially unstable plaque at risk of rupturing and abruptly blocking the coronary artery, which is often the precipitating event in a heart attack; and for neural imaging, particularly in kids, since the portable equipment fits in a helmet, which is far easier than trying to get some wild child to lay still in an MRI scanner.

There are all sorts of other weird and wonderful imaging techniques in development. Elastography, tactile photacoustic imaging, and thermography spring to mind, for example. Fantastic advances in imaging with scopes, robots, swallowed pills, and other natty devices are being made, too.

It's a race to see who can devise the most effective, safest, most mobile, versatile, cheapest imaging device. And to see who can make the first real tricorder.

OTHER DIAGNOSTIC STUFF

Imaging is just one way of exploring the human body and its pathologies. Evolution and miniaturization of computers, electronics, and bioengineering have facilitated wild and wonderful advances in other fields. Advances leading to sensing devices that monitor biochemical and bodily functions down to a cellular level, and sometimes allowing highly localized treatment.

Gene activation microchips, sometimes called DNA microarrays, are one example that sounds so fantastic, it must surely be the stuff of some science fiction writer's fertile imagination. But it's becoming a reality.

They contain probes that can tell which genes within a cell are active and forewarn if something's going wrong. Once we connect this technology to some kind of warning system, we'll be up to speed with our cars and their "check engine" indicator lights.

Or, to move beyond mere sensing, "Eventually scientists will be able to model and mold the incredibly complex interaction between genes and the environment that determines physical and mental health or disease over the life span," predicts Robert E. Adler, Ph.D, in *Medical Firsts: From Hippocrates to the Human Genome.*

Advances in immunology have allowed development of a combination of antibodies and magnetic beads that can detect/diagnose single cancer cells among billions of blood cells in circulation, or donor DNA in a transplant recipient experiencing organ rejection.

Other monitoring seems to verge on the bizarre. There are contact lenses that change color and tattoos that fluoresce in proportion to blood sugar levels (surely an enhancement to any goth or punk getup).

Evolution of microbots, or tiny robots no thicker than a few strands of hair and one-quarter mm long, is another innovation from the realm of the fantastic. They can be injected to gather information and images, and in the future, they'll deliver drugs and perform small operations, like unblocking blood vessels.

At Monash University in Australia, researchers are working on these microbots, taking their inspiration from Hollywood. They're developing a tiny self-propelled robot (driven by a whip like tail mimicking flagellate bacteria) named Proteus, after the vehicle in Fantastic Voyage. The only thing missing is a minaturized Raquel Welch.

Carnegie Mellon University researchers are working on a "pillbot," which are capsules containing a mini camera you swallow. Capsules with cameras aren't new, but previously they've been passively propelled by normal peristaltic action. This left them subject to the whims of where, and how fast, the GI tract carries them. This device propels itself to formerly inaccessible spots and should soon be capable of delivering medicines, taking biopsies, and cauterizing bleeding points.

Other interesting ingestable and implantable gizmos help people comply with prescriptions.

If you forget to take your medicine, pill organizers with alarms can alert you or your doctor. But more sophisticated tattletale pills developed by the University of Florida engineering department contain a miniscule antennae and microchip that signals to an external device that the pill has been taken.

The last patient I saw who would benefit from this was so amnesic he didn't even remember being carted off to the ER after the last seizure, which happened because he didn't remember to take his medicines, had no money or insurance and lived in a tent on the outskirts of town. I doubt he'd be able to afford anything as fancy as this, but let's not tarnish the wonders of innovation with depressing realities.

Implantable devices can administer your medicine. There's the contraceptive chip, for example, manufactured by MicroCHIPS. It uses an electric current to release contraceptive hormones at intervals over a sixteen-year period. It can be turned on or off with a sensor placed over it on the skin, which could be a real boon in the

Third World, though there are some anxieties about unauthorized "hackers" turning fertility on or off.

THE SMARTEST OF SMARTPHONES

These minaturized computers called smartphones have taken over our lives and are finding utility in diagnosis and patient monitoring and management. Welcome to the age of mobile health, or mHealth.

As of this writing, about 75 percent of cell phone users and 80 percent of doctors have smartphones. *The Economist* claims smartphones have "made a bigger difference to the lives of more people, more quickly, than any other technology."

Some medical uses require nothing more than standard features. Others need some sort of attachment that uses the phone as a platform for display or sound.

Doctors are now prescribing apps that help patients manage their conditions. DiabetesManager, developed by WellDoc, analyzes blood sugar, diet, and medicines and gives advice, for instance. *The New York Times* reports it "was show to reduce significantly the blood sugar levels in diabetes patients."

One inventive doctor from the University of Southern Arizona's Limb Salvage Alliance used FaceTime not to see the smiling face of his colleague (whose input he wanted, but who was away at a conference), but to show him the foot wound of a diabetic patient he was worried about.

Many gizmos and apps can assist your doctor. He can turn his smartphone into an electronic stethoscope, as with the Thinklabs ds32a+ digital stethoscope. It comes with an app that tells him much more about your heart than he ever knew before (or wanted to know?).

Phones can take "hospital quality" ECGs with SmartHeart, which attaches with a strap around your chest, or with CardioDefender, which attaches as a wristband. Add an ultrasound probe and you can display ultrasound images. And recently, the FDA approved the Mobile MIM, the first mobile radiology application where CTs, MRIs, PET scans, and the like can be read on an iPhone or iPad.

With the right sensor, smartphones monitor vital signs and blood oxygen levels. Or, for pregnant women and women in labor, the AirStripOB is one of several devices that attach to the skin, sort of like a glorified BandAid, to monitor uterine and fetal heart activity.

Other sensors and attachments—not necessarily in conjunction with smartphones—monitor for pressure sores or balance, while others positively identify patients when administering drugs or track their movements. The latter is helpful with wandering patients in nursing homes/dementia units and newborn nurseries to stop abductions, for example.

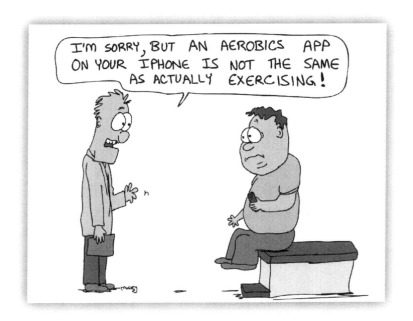

Biochemical And STIs

With the help of miniaturized pathology lab technology, diabetics can measure blood glucose and hemoglobin A1c, patients on anticoagulants can monitor pro time, and even things like circulating allergens and tumor markers can be measured. The iBG-Star, made by insulin-producing drug company Sanofi, "tracks your glucose, carbohydrate intake, and the dosage of insulin that should be administered." No surprise that Sanofi presumes insulin use.

For the amorous—especially those who'd rather not show their faces in the sexually transmitted infections clinic—Dr. Tariq Sadiq, senior lecturer and consultant physician in sexual health and HIV, and his team at St. George's University of London created the eSTI 2. An app and phone attachment diagnose STIs (the preferred term for STDs) from a drop of urine or saliva.

The *New York Observer* suggests the true utility: rather than finding out after the fact, test your potential consort "and then decide whether or not to 'finish the download'."

Or, for a more touchy-feely test, check the emotional status of your partner. Companies like Cogito Health and "affective computing" make it possible by monitoring the speed and accuracy of typing, how much the phone shakes, and phone manner.

The Third World

Some innovations are less utilitarian for party animals in the industrialized world, but are becoming a real boon to medical care in Third World countries.

Cheap phones like the Ideos XI Android, made by Huawei, sells for $80 in Kenya. Combined with something like MedKenya, which the MobileHealthNews website describes as "a reference app similar to WebMD" that "provides symptom checkers, first aid information, medical alerts, and searchable doctor and hospital directories," this can be invaluable to large underserved rural populations. Of course, there are parts of the U.S. that could do with something like this too.

Specialized apps like LifeLens detect malaria in a picture of a blood sample taken with a phone. NETRA (Near-Eye Tool for Refractive Assessment), developed by Camera Culture MIT

Media, uses a special phone screen to do an instant refraction for eyeglasses.

But don't expect any great innovation to go unregulated. Medical apps are receiving scrutiny as medical devices by the FDA, and this worries some people. They're not so excited about apps that monitor your health habits like diet, exercise, weight, and sleep. A September 2013 report by CBS News notes, "The FDA will be concentrating on regulating mobile medical apps that are intended to be used as an accessory to an already-regulated medical device," like an ultrasound or electrocardiogram. There is concern that the cost and the FDA's glacial approval pace will stifle the medical apps industry currently evolving at a frenetic pace.

One real boon is that doctors no longer have to be stuck in the hospital or office or connected to a land line. It's certainly not like the old days, when one slightly goofy but ingenious doc in my group kept a quarter taped to his pager so he could always use a pay phone if he got an urgent page on the road. Increased mobility means the doctor can monitor and interact with patients from anywhere, even the golf course.

DETECTION AND TREATMENT: THE CLOSED LOOP

Another concept coming into fruition is the idea of the closed loop, a halfway house between assessment and treatment, where sensing what's wrong is tied to treatment.

Diabetes is again a good example. Many innovations are directed at diabetes, and appropriately so, with the storm clouds of the obesity and diabetes epidemic building. If your blood sugar monitoring system is tied directly to your insulin pump, you can mimic the responses your pancreas should be making.

Systems are also in development to detect nucleic acid in the blood released in unstable angina (the harbinger of a heart attack). They can release anti-inflammatory and anti-clotting medicines to instantly reduce the risk of having an attack.

Like DNA probes, microbots, and other marvels, "This closed loop sensing-and-dosing model may seem far fetched," says Topol, but "the technical capabilities exist today."

TREATMENT FROM THE FUTURE

Genomics and these very sophisticated sensing mechanisms are getting better and better at telling us what's wrong. But then we have to do something about it. Or, better still, move into predict-and-prevent mode to stop problems from happening in the first place.

IMMUNIZATION

Immunization is the ultimate in predict-and-prevent medicine, though there has been "lack of attention and priority for vaccine development," laments Topol. The U.S. healthcare system currently tends to pay much more attention to treatment than prevention.

"Immunization" is the preferred word, note the fastidious wordsmiths. We're moving away from "vaccine," with its Latin meaning of cows and associated images of Edward Jenner inoculating milkmaids with pus from cowpox-infected udder sores.

Newer uses of immunization are in cancer management. They prevent infections that predispose to cancer, as with Gardasil to protect [hopefully] not yet sexually active tweens against cervical cancer-causing human papilloma virus (HPV), or immunizing against Hepatitis B, which is the most common cause of liver cancer worldwide.

The real cutting-edge stuff uses proteins derived from cancers to induce an immune response to the tumor. Provenge, the first and only FDA-approved product for personalized immunotherapy for advanced prostate cancer, as the website boasts, is a good example.

Components from the prostate cancer are used to sensitize immune cells in the lab, which are then reintroduced to seek out and destroy the cancer cells, kind of like giving hounds the scent of a fox.

There's speculation that some illnesses we do not currently think of as infections may in fact be so, and thus be preventable with immunization. Maverick Australian researcher Barry Marshall shook up the world by doing what any self-respecting researcher would do to prove his point: inoculating himself by drinking a *Helicobacter pylori* culture, thus proving infection with this organism causes peptic ulcers.

Now researchers are postulating Alzheimer's and atheroma may be caused by infections, and that herpes simplex type 2

(HSV2, which causes genital herpes) may play some role in bipolar disorder and schizophrenia.

COMPUTERS AND ROBOTS IN YOUR FUTURE

As computers and computer-controlled robotics develop and become more refined, their medical applications are quickly increasing, far beyond electronic health records and smartphones.

SURGERY

I think of most surgery as a failure of medical prevention/treatment to keep the patient away from some knife-wielding handyman intent on putting something in or taking something out. Still, that doesn't undermine the iconic image of a group of heroic surgeons in gowns with shiny instruments clustered around, dismembering some prostrate person. The real heroes are, of course, the rumpled, dowdy primary care doctors in their mismatched tweeds and shabby offices, skillfully keeping patients out of the hands of the surgeon.

But surgery is, for the moment, an irrefutable part of healthcare, and it's evolving. Conventional surgery is being increasingly replaced by minimally invasive "keyhole" surgery, with tools like laparoscopes, arthroscopes, thoracoscopes, culposcopes, and colonoscopes, through which surgeons can somehow remove the gall bladder, stomach, lung, appendix, kidney, or other part with nothing more than one or two small stab wounds. This translates to far less pain, morbidity, scarring, risk of infection, and faster recovery.

Another refinement, NOTES (Natural Orifice Transluminal Endoscopic Surgery), refers to surgery performed directly through the orifices that god put there. For example, removing the gall bladder through the mouth or appendix through the vagina, thus avoiding stab wounds altogether.

The real cutting-edge stuff is with computer-controlled robotics like the da Vinci system. The operator sits at a control console while the "patient-side cart," which is immune to things like fatigue, distraction, and backache that limit mere mortals, does the surgery. With its three arms, highly flexible wrists, and a 3D camera, it enhances the skills of any surgeon.

With such systems, all movements are transmitted through and modulated by the computer (eliminating any clumsiness or tremor the surgeon might suffer from that bender the night before). Plus, the operator doesn't have to be on site, but can be anywhere with a computer hookup and the requisite machinery.

All the way back in 2001, Dr. Jacques Marescaux removed the gall bladder of a 68-year-old patient in Strasbourg, France from New York. Dr. Anvari, a surgeon in Hamilton, Canada, has conducted numerous remote surgeries on patients in North Bay, a city 250 miles away.

Robotic surgery is also encroaching into orthopedics, where, with the help of 3D imaging from CT or MRI scans, it's particularly good at relocating bone fragments from bad fractures.

Further, like our smartphones with Siri, surgical robots can be controlled by voice commands. Italian surgeon Carlo

Pappone is pushing the boundaries even further, using an autonomous robot operating from information stored from previous procedures. Such robots have already performed relatively simple heart surgery to ablate aberrant electrical pathways in patients with atrial fibrillation.

Makers of the da Vinci system obviously worry about people thinking independent robots are going to muscle the surgeon aside and take over. They stress their creation operates on a "master/slave" relationship, offering assurances that the surgeon is the master.

This remote presence technology is of interest to the military. The June 2009 *International Journal of Medical Robotics* reports on a rapidly deployed robotic system that can insert IVs, intubate to provide an airway, perform nursing duties, and complete simple operations to stabilize the patient "autonomously or in a teleoperative mode on wounded soldiers in the battlefield who might otherwise die before treatment in a combat hospital could be provided."

Part of the technology and impetus for surgical robotics has come from an industry you might see as more focused on death and violence than repair and saving lives: gaming. There is cross-pollination going on, with surgical and medical applications feeding off game industry developments.

Purdue University is developing a robotic scrub nurse who responds to hand signals as newer game consoles like Wii do. The University of Washington is using Microsoft's Kinect (launched in America in November 2010, taking the Guinness World Record for fastest-selling consumer electronics device) and the Xbox 360 to give surgeons tactile information about the field he's operating on (like by making the control stick lock if the surgeon hits something solid like bone). It similarly allows programming of "no-fly zones" to keep the surgeon away from vital organs like nerves, blood vessels, ureters, and other things they sometimes nick with sharp instruments with disastrous consequences.

The ability for a surgeon to be remote, perhaps comfortable in his home office, from a patient, possibly lying on a battlefield in Afghanistan, is attractive. The main catch is that the remote location be properly equipped with the right machinery, connections, and security (I wouldn't want someone hacking the system in the middle of my operation).

One other interesting, particularly modern-day American problem, is the question of liability. When the robot operating on you screws up, whom do you sue?

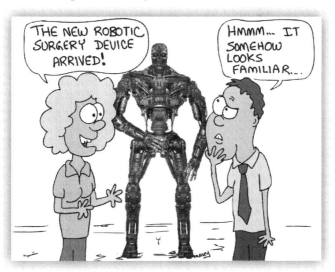

Superseding Surgery

Surgeons aren't just being threatened by robots these days. They're also losing ground to interventional radiologists.

The ability of specialized radiologists to stick needles, stents, catheters, electrodes, and other hardware pretty much anywhere in the body—all with the unfair advantage of X-ray or ultrasound guidance—allows many conditions to be treated without any cutting.

Unblocking blood vessels is one of the more successful applications. The technique was pioneered by 1978 Nobel Prize nominee Charles Dotter, M.D., who opened a blocked artery in the leg of an 82-year-old woman with a "gangrene-ravaged left foot," according to the Society of Interventional Radiology website.

"To her surgeon's disbelief, her pain ceased, she started walking, and three 'irreversibly' gangrenous toes spontaneously sloughed. She left the hospital on both feet."

Whether they're obstructed by a clot or plaque buildup, it's often possible to unblock a blood vessel with a balloon, stent, or thrombolytic medicines to dissolve any blood clot and restore circulation.

Sometimes, you want to do the opposite. For troublesome peptic ulcers or tumors that keep bleeding, interventional radiologists can embolize a blood vessel, deliberately causing the blood to clot and cutting off the blood supply.

In other illnesses, they can use invasive techniques to locally administer cryotherapy, radio frequency ablation, or a host of medicines to precisely wipe out unwanted tissues, such as cancers.

Watching interventional radiologists maneuvering their gadgets and zapping the bad guys always looks like some kind of a computer game to me (and, as noted, that may be how it started). Combined with the fabulous reimbursement in our insane payment system for any kind of procedure, it's no wonder all the young bucks in medical school want to be interventional radiologists, rather than some harassed, downtrodden, underpaid primary care doctor.

SIMULATORS

Robotic simulators help train surgeons and other healthcare personnel. The increasing sophistication of the computers controlling these simulators makes them ever more lifelike in the conditions they mimic.

It's a nice idea that a surgeon can practice and work out his kinks on a robot rather than you. That's now possible through a training program with the International College of Robotic Surgery. Even if some gung-ho surgeon can't wait to get to the real thing, the FDA safeguards by mandating training on robots before certain procedures, like the increasingly popular placing of stents in the carotid arteries in the neck to prevent strokes.

The practice manikins for nurses, medical students, EMTs, firefighters, and others are also becoming more sophisticated. For example, their hearts are controlled by computers that mimic abnormal rhythms, they have tricky airways for more realistic intubation, and they have synthetic veins to practice putting in

IVs. There's even "Fat Old Fred," a bariatric manikin for students who "wonder how CPR manikins will compare with real victims," notes the manufacturer at first-aid-products.com.

REMOTE PRESENCE

As noted, remote presence allows doctors and surgeons to communicate with and operate on people somewhere else. Robotics are being developed to make this a more everyday occurrence.

RP-VITA (Remote Presence Virtual + Independent Telemedicine Assistant) is a self-propelled robot programmed to do rounds and visit patients in the hospital. It features an interactive video screen, the ability to gather and transmit vital sign data, and its own stethoscope.

Who needs a doctor?

Despite waggish touches, like dressing these robots in white coats, I cannot help but wonder—when patients in the office are already disturbed by doctors ignoring them in favor of the computer—how will they react when R2-D2 glides to the bedside and inquires after their health in a Dalek voice?

But, "The robot is remarkably personal. It provides virtual communication and patients really like him," says Garth H. Ballantyne, M.D., of Hackensack University Medical Center, where they've been using a similar robot called "Mr. Rounder."

Remote presence technology can also provide helpful communication from doctor to doctor.

I did a locum tenens in an isolated, rinky-dink prairie town in Saskatchewan (it may be overstating things to call it a town). An old farmer with some kind of hepatitis (there were no records) had his tractor or some piece of equipment fall on him. His family brought him in all in a panic. He was in pain, he looked pretty gray, his blood pressure was low, and he was tender all down the right side of his abdomen, which seemed bloated. He had a low-grade fever, his chest X-ray looked a little hazy, and his blood work showed a little anemia and a slightly elevated white blood cell count.

I was nonplussed. I didn't know whether to transfuse him, give him antibiotics, give him pain medicine (and risk masking the symptoms of an acute abdomen), or tap his abdomen to check for blood or fluid.

We packed him in the local ambulance, a decrepit fourth-generation Chrysler Town and Country, for a bumpy 90-mile ride to Regina, the nearest place with a reasonable-sized hospital. I found out later he had a right side empyema (an infection in the pleural cavity), and the accident probably had very little to do with his illness.

I remember thinking at the time, "There are people who would know what to do much better than me. They just don't happen to be here."

I could have done with a system like the one provided by a company called VISCU and pioneered by Dr. Michael Breslow. It's a call center staffed 24/7 by intensivists (intensive care specialists) who monitor patients in multiple ICUs and dispense advice.

A similar program, started in Idaho, allows obstetricians from peripheral hospitals to consult with neonatologist regarding premature babies. This facilitates the start of appropriate treatments even before transport to a more suitable location.

Another variation is a specially equipped ambulance in Germany, the VIMED STEMO, which has a CT scanner on board, "integrates a fully functioning pre-clinical stroke care suite, comparable to those found in specialized stroke hospitals," and can send encrypted information to ERs or trauma centers "for nearly instant diagnosis and initiation of treatment." The maxim in stroke treatment these days is "Time is brain;" if it's an ischemic stroke with an artery blocked by thrombus, clot-buster medicine should be started ASAP.

SOME ELECTRIFYING TREATMENTS

Electronics advances are particularly benefiting the field of neurology. Techniques are being developed to either apply electrical stimulation or to detect and use the electric currents our nerves generate.

Deep brain stimulation provides tiny electrical impulses to the brain or nerves from a pulse generator implanted under the chest skin or abdominal wall via leads inserted into the brain (under local anesthetic, but with the patient awake). It has shown promise controlling the tremor of patients with Parkinson's, and at Ohio State University, researchers have been trying it for Alzheimer's.

It also seems capable of modifying aberrant behaviors, like Tourette's syndrome outbursts or—in what might sound like something Stephen King would write—it's been tried for changing what some classify as character flaws, like obsessive-compulsive disorder.

Topol relates the case of a severely depressed, near-catatonic man who'd been an inpatient for years and was totally devoid of emotion who was treated with deep brain stimulation. The neurosurgeons fished around until they found a spot that, when stimulated, made the man smile for the first time in years. When connected to the pulse generator, the patient became a totally different person, affable, friendly, and able to be discharged.

Unfortunately, his affability took an overzealous turn. His wife called a few days later, complaining the patient, who'd been sexually inactive for fifteen years, now "wanted to have sex continuously."

Also, stimulating the vagus nerve with electrodes implanted in the neck is a mechanism being developed to reduce or prevent seizures.

Then there's transcranial magnetic stimulation, generating tiny electrical currents in the brain. An advantage is that nothing has to be stuck in your brain; instead, magnetic coils are applied to the exterior of your head (I can't help picturing this done in some dungeon by Gene Wilder). Originally, this was used for mapping areas of brain activity, but the electric currents generated seem able to treat various psychiatric diseases, and it's recently been tried for migraines.

Or, rather than administering electrical impulses, these sophisticated electronics systems and inserted electrodes can pick up the tiny electrical currents generated by nerves, muscles, or brain and use them to activate robotic devices.

A team at Massachusetts General Hospital recently reported in *Nature* on their "Brain Gate" system. A woman paralyzed for fifteen years was able to activate a robot with her thoughts and use it to lift a bottle to her lips so she could drink out of it using a straw.

Perhaps most impressive was Zac Vawter, a 31-year-old amputee who climbed 103 floors to the top of the Willis Tower, America's tallest skyscraper, on a thought-activated prosthetic leg.

Chalmers University of Technology in Sweden fitted a 42-year-old amputee with a new arm, also controlled by the patient's mind, but that they claim also operates well enough for him to go back to work as a truck driver and tie his shoe laces.

The best power-to-the-people medical emancipation story of electronic-activated prostheses is that of 6-year-old Alex Pring, one of some 1,500 kids born each year missing part of his arm or hand. He provided a challenge for a University of Central Florida engineering group specializing in prostheses who've named themselves "Limbitless." They manufactured a robotic arm for Alex with a 3D printer out of off-the-shelf servos and batteries; it's activated by Alex's biceps muscles and only cost $350.

ORGANIZATIONAL FUTURE

The future of healthcare isn't all computers, microelectronics, gadgets, and gizmos. Some of it is logistical and organizational changes, much of which I touch on in different chapters throughout.

Doctors' offices are changing. They are being taken over by corporations, with the trend to turn them into widget factories with a close eye on productivity, often making your relationship with your doctor less personal and visits more time pressured. Sometimes you don't get to see your doctor at all, but only an extender. Computers are changing the organization (often for the better), but they may interpose between you and your doctor.

Different reimbursement models are likely to incentivize prevention, encouraged by the Affordable Care Act. This legislation also brings many innovations of its own, of course, like expanded Medicaid, eliminating prohibitions on preexisting conditions, removing lifetime caps on coverage, expanding coverage for young adults, preventive services without co-payment or deductibles, incentives for accountable care organizations, increasing the relative remuneration of primary care, mandatory electronic health records, and much more.

But most significant to you, who must have a serious interest in being a self-sufficient patient if you've read this far, is the massive increase in the availability of information and the expansion of emancipation-friendly providers, whether allopathic or complementary and alternative.

IN CLOSING

I picked what I think are some of the most significant changes and innovations taking place in healthcare. But changes and innovations are exploding all across the broad field of medicine, which is going through its very own Big Bang. This makes it impossible to touch on all of it or even to pick out the most significant stuff, or to keep everything current in a print format.

But I hope it's been interesting and, more importantly, that it might help steer you and your doctor toward options neither of you may have otherwise been aware of.

CHAPTER 8

MEDICAL KIT

———◆———

LIVE LIKE AN AUSSIE

I've seen no more rugged, self-sufficient, medically emancipated people than those working the cattle and sheep "stations" in the Australian Outback. They live in what Bill Bryson called "a sunburned country," where the nearest neighbor may be 200 miles away. Their independence is greatly aided by comprehensive medical kits.

I had the chance to see this emancipation in action during a stint in the Royal Flying Doctor Service (RFDS) out of Broken Hill, a rough, tough mining town in the very heart of the Australia.

Each station had a kit with standard medicines the doctor could prescribe, as well as dressings and other equipment (including a bladder catheter, which left me wondering how anyone would fare using it, even with instructions over the radio link that connected every station to the RFDS base).

As the name implies, doctors had to fly massive distances to see sick patients or hold clinics, often on hot, dusty verandas. The radio was an integral part of what Reverend John Flynn, founder of the service, called "the mantle of safety." It served other purposes too, including afternoon chat sessions in which isolated farmers' wives usually participated. These were chauvinistically referred to as "galah sessions," so-named for the raucous squawking of the native galah cockatoos.

On-air "clinics" were conducted twice daily, though the fact that everyone could listen in prompted some reluctance to consult about weeping genital sores or the old man's drinking problem. Anyone could call any time and talk to the doctor, which oddly gave these isolated folks better access than people have in "the civilized world."

You can greatly enhance your independence by taking a cue from the RFDS playbook and having some medical equipment and drugs at home. After all, it's the ultimate medical emancipation when you don't even have to involve a doctor.

It can also help you save money by letting you pick cheap medicines, like store generic brands, instead of some expensive name brand the doctor chooses.

Your ideal medical kit contents depend on how adventurous and informed you are, and possibly on your particular conditions. Remember, I'm not advising you about what to take on an expedition to the Amazon—just what I recommend the average household have around. So, I'm not including IVs, sutures, anesthetics, or bladder catheters. Some medicines require a prescription, and therefore your doctor's cooperation.

THE RIGHT MEDS

As for medicines, the best approach is probably to talk about specific symptoms/ailments and what drugs will help (and how). Remember, most medicines have a generic name and one or more brand names.

RESPIRATORY

The most common ailment in this category is congestion/inflammation of the respiratory tract, with symptoms like sore throat, blocked or running nose, sinus or ear congestion, and cough.

If all this is due to an infection, as with a cold (or URI, an upper respiratory infection, to use the proper jargon), the virus may also give you a low-grade fever for the first day or so (likely in the 99 to 101 degrees Fahrenheit range). Allergies can present a similar picture, and there are various other causes.

Countless URI medicines are available with combinations of a few specific ingredients, so look for the product containing the active ingredient(s) you want at the lowest price.

Guaifenesin is an expectorant in many URI treatments. It thins the mucus and makes your sinus, ears, and nose drain better, and makes mucus in your chest easier to get up when you cough.

Antihistamines help dry up a runny nose and have a specific benefit for allergies. The problem is so-called "first generation" ones like diphenhydramine, chlorpheniramine, and brompheniramine usually make people drowsy (so are used in OTC sleep aids). If you prefer to avoid this effect, splurge on a more expensive second-generation non-sedating antihistamine like cetirizine or loratidine.

Decongestants like pseudoephedrine and phenylephrine, which are in many of the "D" decongestant products, also help unblock your nose and sinuses, but may elevate your blood pressure or pulse rate, so watch out if you have heart or vascular disease.

OTC nose sprays with oxymetazoline are good for quickly unblocking your nose (and sticking a cotton ball soaked in it up your nose is a great way to stop a nose bleed). The disadvantage is that if you use one of these for days on end, your nose gets "addicted" and develops rebound congestion without it.

For a cough, dextromethorphan is an appropriate cough suppressant. It's not as strong as codeine, but you need a prescription for codeine as it's one of those wicked opiates that dull not only your cough, but also your pain and your brain and turn you in to a raving addict if you're not careful. Or that's the fear at the FDA, at least.

Lots of home/natural remedies for URIs make use of stuff like cinnamon, chamomile, lemon, honey, and cayenne pepper, or call for flushing out your nose and sinuses with a Neti pot. You may prefer this approach to all these "white-man medicines," but I don't know a whole lot about them and consider them beyond the scope of what I'm telling you here. Do your research.

If you're susceptible to an asthmatic sort of reaction to lung irritation, getting tight, wheezy, and short of breath, a bronchodilator helps relieve these symptoms.

Racemic epinephrine in Asthmanefrin, used with an EZ Breathe atomizer, is a fairly new—and pricey—OTC inhaler (which the FDA worries may be harmful to people with heart disease). There's also OTC ephedrine/guafenasin in Primatene tablets (there used to be a Primatene mist inhaler, but it was withdrawn because the CFC propellants are undesirable).

Many prescription inhalers tend to have less side effects, the most common being albuterol. And remember, asthma is potentially fatal. There are more than 3,300 related deaths per year, many preventable, so when in doubt, get help.

GASTROINTESTINAL

The next most common ailment is GI upset. Of these, the most urgent is gastroenteritis or a "stomach bug," with symptoms like nausea, vomiting, abdominal pain, bloating, and diarrhea, which in the early stages can be profuse and watery ("the squirts," as it is sometimes charmingly referred to). This too is usually caused by a viral infection, though occasionally it's bacterial (especially when traveling in the Third World). Toxins in spoiled food can cause the same kind of symptoms.

Any first generation antihistamine will help with nausea, even if it's from some other cause like motion sickness. Emetrol is a combination of fructose, dextrose, and phosphoric acid that soothes the stomach.

For help at the other end, loperamide (which is in Imodium) slows down diarrhea and reduces cramps to some extent. It does nothing to get rid of the infection, remember; it just makes life a little more bearable. It can be a life saver if you're doing game parks on a tour bus in Kenya, for example, as on a trip I took with my first wife, when everyone got "tourista" and was pleading with the driver to stop every five minutes.

Time is usually what gets rid of the infection, helped along by eating light and replenishing your fluids and electrolytes. Gatorade is good for this, or make your own oral rehydration fluid with ½ to 1 teaspoon of salt and 6 teaspoons of sugar per liter or quart of water.

Dyspepsia/heartburn is another common malady it's nice to have a treatment for. The most basic is with antacids containing calcium carbonate as the principal ingredient, like Tums and Rolaids. At the next level are H2 blockers like ranitidine (Zantac) and famotidine (Pepcid) or proton pump inhibitors (PPIs) like omeprazole (Prilosec) and lansoprazole (Prevacid).

Be aware that alcohol, smoking, spicy and acidic foods, and NSAIDs are particularly irritating to your stomach.

Pain And Fever

Multiple pain medicines are available over the counter. The biggest group is non-steroidal anti-inflammatory drugs (NSAIDs), which includes ibuprofen, naproxen, and aspirin. As the name suggests, they have an anti-inflammatory effect, so they're good for arthritis, sprains, and inflamed tendons and muscles (though aspirin has only mild pain-relieving and anti-inflammatory effects).

Acetaminophen (the ingredient in—and just about synonymous with—Tylenol, a testament to McNeil Pharmaceutical's marketing prowess) is another common pain reliever, but it isn't an NSAID. It has no anti-inflammatory effect, and it's less irritating on the stomach than NSAIDs.

Both acetaminophen and NSAIDs reduce a fever. Keep in mind, though, that fevers may help your body fight infection, so treating a low one isn't necessarily always the best tactic. But fevers also makes you feel like crap, so most people treat them.

There seems to be a lot of anxiety about NSAIDs being rough on the liver and/or kidneys lately, which I think is putting people off unnecessarily. This mostly seems to be a concern for people with existing liver or kidney problems. NSAIDs work a bit like salt on your heart and blood pressure, so if you have heart disease or hypertension, be careful.

There's also concern about acetaminophen being harmful to the liver, which again I think is exaggerated. The maximum dose is 1 gram (1000 mg, and it comes in many different strengths, but usually 325, 500, or 650 mg) every four hours, or no more than 4 grams per day. Overdose of acetaminophen is very toxic to the liver.

NSAIDs and acetaminophen aren't very strong pain killers. It's not a bad idea to have a few stronger pain meds at home in case you break your leg or something. But most of the strong pain meds are opiates like codeine, so they require a prescription and the trust of your doctor (as noted above, it's the same codeine that's in strong cough medicines, a fact put to good use on a mission trip to Haiti when I needed to clean the raw burns of a child and had no anesthetic—except a bottle of cough medicine).

Dental pain can be one of the most troublesome. Treat it like any other pain. I was brought up on oil of cloves, which you paint on the tooth to numb it, and there are oral anesthetics like Orabase.

Topical Medicines

Topical medicines are applied locally to the problem. Many are helpful to have on hand.

Skin creams or ointments (ointments are oil based, so they're greasier but longer lasting) with hydrocortisone (you can get up to 1 percent solutions over the counter) are good for irritated skin (including from a sunburn) and itchy rashes. Calamine lotion is a traditional skin-soothing potion.

Eye drops with tetrahydrozoline (as in Visine) reduce redness and irritation. Lubricant drops made with glycerin or propylene glycol are also good for irritated eyes.

Some treatment for swimmer's ear (which is really a water-induced dermatitis of the ear canal) is worth stocking if you swim. Medicines that treat established swimmers ear are by prescription, but isopropyl alcohol drops (used in products like Auro-Dri to prevent the problem) dry out the ear canal and may well work. However, putting alcohol on any inflamed surface, including your ear canal, can be pretty uncomfortable.

Antiseptic/antibiotic ointments containing chlorhexidine or combinations of neomycin, bacitracin, polymyxin B, and pramoxine are good for treating or preventing skin infections. These are often used together with dressings (see below).

It's smart to have something for treating burns. A cream containing silver sulfadiazine is appropriate, but it requires a prescription. Topical antiseptics/antibiotics are a second choice.

The maddening condition that's the butt of so many jokes—hemorrhoids—can be treated with a multitude of different ingredients like witch hazel, hydrocortisone, and pramoxine. Use them in ointment form, or to get to those upper reaches, in suppositories.

MISCELLANEOUS

Any home medical kit should include an ample selection of various sizes of adhesive bandage strips (like Band-Aids), gauze squares, and non-adherent dressings for wounds. Cleaning wounds with hydrogen peroxide and applying a topical antiseptic/antibiotic under the dressing is important for preventing infections.

Alcohol wipes are also useful for cleaning small areas of skin, while hand sanitizers help you avoid contaminating a wound while tending to it. Sterile gloves work too.

Bandages (especially self-adhesive ones) and slings help manage sprains and sore, inflamed joints.

Superglue is a useful new addition for closing small cuts and cracks in dry skin. They're increasingly using a fancy version of it in hospitals and ERs.

As for hardware, fine non-toothed forceps are useful for lots of things, including removing splinters. A measuring cup, thermometer, flashlight, sunscreen, insect repellant, safety pins, scissors, water filter or purifying tablets, and a space blanket can all come in handy, especially if you're traveling.

They say a set of car keys is the most essential first aid item for anyone with a snakebite, so you or someone can drive to the hospital ASAP. Heroics like tourniquets and sucking out the poison aren't really effective; you need antivenom if it's poisonous.

One slightly controversial item that's a real boon in the right circumstances is a course of broad-spectrum antibiotic like azithromycin or levofloxacin. This requires a prescription from your doctor. It's controversial in that you really need to know if it's appropriate for the particular infection, which even doctors have trouble figuring out sometimes. Antibiotics are for bacterial infections, and each class has its strong and weak points when it comes to fighting different strains of bacteria. Overuse and inappropriate use of antibiotics, as I talked about earlier, has been causing some problems.

Still, for bacterial infections like pneumonia, sinusitis, ear infections, bacterial gastroenteritis, UTIs, wound infections, and a whole lot more, nipping it in the bud without waiting to get to the doctor for a prescription can make a big difference.

To belabor a point about antibiotics that many people have tried to make, but which seems very hard to get across, is that URIs in early stages cannot be treated with antibiotics. Sometimes a secondary sinus or ear infection or bronchitis justifies antibiotics, but usually only if it's at least two to three weeks later.

Another controversial idea that requires a prescription is carrying some kind of basic anxiety medicine like alprazolam, diazepam, or clonazepam for when you're getting totally stressed out about something. Medicines like this also make you sleepy, which is helpful for long flights.

If you take maintenance medicines, put a few days' supply in your carry-on for when the airline loses your checked baggage or some other mishap strikes. On long trips, keep things like pain or motion sickness medicines close at hand.

Activated charcoal for treating poisonings and ipecac to induce vomiting are other things to consider keeping in your kit. However, both are a bit iffy and ideally should only be used under medical supervision. For poisoning emergencies, consult a poison help center, like the National Capital Poison Center at 1-800-222-1222 (www.poison.org).

Depending on your circumstances and personal health, consider specialized inclusions. For example, if you or someone in your household has life-threatening allergies, get a prescription for an epinephrine auto-injector like an EpiPen or Twinject.

Include a list of contacts with phone numbers for when you're beyond the realm of DIY treatment. This would include your G.P. and specialists, plus numbers for the hospital, ambulance, poison control center, and personal emergency contacts. Add in your medical history and consent forms, a simple note explaining any special medical conditions or needs, and a copy of your advance directive.

12|15

Orange County Library System
146A Madison Rd.
Orange, VA 22960
(540) 672-3811 www.ocplva.org

Made in the USA
Charleston, SC
05 October 2015